TheraSci User's Guide

Thera*Scribe*® User's Guide

For use with:
- Thera*Scribe*® 5.0 Small Practice Edition
- Thera*Scribe*® 5.0 Enterprise Edition
- Thera*Scribe*® Essential 1.0

Arthur E. Jongsma, Jr., PhD, and PEC Technologies

John Wiley & Sons, Inc.

This text is printed on acid-free paper. ∞

Copyright © 2007 by Arthur E. Jongsma, Jr. All rights reserved.
Published by John Wiley & Sons, Inc.
Published simultaneously in Canada

Wiley Bicentennial Logo: Richard J. Pacifico

Designations used by companies to distinguish their products are often claimed as trademarks. In all instances where John Wiley & Sons, Inc. is aware of a claim, the product names appear in initial capital or all capital letters in this text. Readers, however, should contact the appropriate companies for more complete information regarding trademarks and registration.

Microsoft Access ®, Microsoft Word ®, and Microsoft Outlook ® are registered trademarks of Microsoft Corporation.
DSM ® and DSM-IV-TR ® are registered trademarks of the American Psychiatric Association.
DSM-IV-TR® codes included in this work are used with the permission of the American Psychiatric Association.
Thera*Scribe* ® is a registered trademark of John Wiley & Sons.

No part of this publication may be reproduced, stored in a retrieval system, or transmitted in any form or by any means, electronic, mechanical, photocopying, recording, scanning, or otherwise, except as permitted under Section 107 or 108 of the 1976 United States Copyright Act, without either the prior written permission of the Publisher, or authorization through payment of the appropriate per-copy fee to the Copyright Clearance Center, 222 Rosewood Drive, Danvers, MA 01923, 978-750-8400, fax 978-646-8400, or on the web at www.copyright.com. Requests to the Publisher for permission should be addressed to the Permissions Department, John Wiley & Sons, Inc., 111 River Street, Hoboken, NJ 07030, 201-748-6011, fax 201-748-6008, or online at http://www.wiley.com/go/permission.

This publication is designed to provide accurate and authoritative information in regard to the subject matter covered. It is sold with the understanding that the publisher is not engaged in rendering professional services. If legal, accounting, medical, psychological, or any other expert assistance is required, the services of a competent professional person should be sought.

THE PURCHASER MAY MAKE BACKUP COPIES FOR HIS/HER OWN USE ONLY AND NOT FOR DISTRIBUTION OR RESALE. THE PUBLISHER ASSUMES NO RESPONSIBILITY FOR ERRORS, OMISSIONS, OR DAMAGES, INCLUDING WITHOUT LIMITATION DAMAGES CAUSED BY THE USE OF THESE FORMS OR FROM THE USE OF THE INFORMATION CONTAINED THEREIN.

ISBN-13 978-0470-00879-9

10 9 8 7 6 5 4 3 2

Contents

Section I—Introduction — 1

Chapter 1 Thera*Scribe*® — 3
- Changes and Enhancements in Thera*Scribe*® 5.0 and Essential 1.0 — 3
- Activation of Thera*Scribe*® — 6
- System Requirements — 7
- Installation — 8

Chapter 2 Feature Overview — 15
- Login — 15
- Home Screen — 17
- File Menu — 18
- Go Menu — 18
- Help Menu — 18
- Navigation Tool Bars — 19
- Types of Fields — 20
- Using Dropdown Lists — 21
- Entering Dates — 22
- Selecting, Adding, and Deleting Patients — 22
- Working with Clinical Pathways — 24
- Selecting from and Editing Libraries — 28
- Screen Customization — 30
- Exiting the System — 34

Section II—Application Screens 35

Chapter 3 Personal Data 37
    Demographics 37
    Provider 39
    Insurance 39
    General Notes 41
    Attachments 41
    Episode Custom Fields 42
    HIPAA 43

Chapter 4 Assessment 45
    Psychosocial History 45
    Strengths/Weaknesses 46
    Assessments Given 47
    Mental Status 50
    Recovery 52
    Summary 54

Chapter 5 Treatment Plan 55
    Problem 56
    Definitions 58
    Goals 59
    Objectives/Interventions 60
    Modality 62
    Approach 64
    Diagnosis 66
    Response 67
    Homework 68

Chapter 6 Progress 71
    Session Details 72
    Progress Notes Planner 74
    Objective Rating 77
    Psychotherapy Notes 78

	Session Custom Fields	78
	Amendments	79

Chapter 7 Prognosis/Discharge — 81
Prognosis Details — 81
Discharge Details — 82

Chapter 8 Appointment Scheduler — 85

Chapter 9 Reports — 89
Clinical Record Reports — 91
Administrative Reports — 95

Chapter 10 Outcomes — 99
Selection Criteria — 100
Results — 102

Chapter 11 Tools — 105
Providers — 106
Teams/Groups — 110
Custom Fields — 111
Default Settings — 111
Shortcut Bar — 112
Libraries — 113
Treatment Planners — 114
Progress Note Planners — 116
Database — 117
System Settings — 126
Preferences — 129

Appendix A Technical Support — 130

Appendix B License Agreement — 131

Index — 134

SECTION I

Introduction

CHAPTER 1
► Thera*Scribe*®

CHAPTER 2
► Feature Overview

Thera*Scribe*® is widely recognized as a powerful, yet easy-to-use, behavioral health treatment planning and clinical record management system. Developed by an experienced clinician, Arthur E. Jongsma, Jr., Ph.D., and a team of knowledgeable programmers at PEC Technologies, Thera*Scribe*® provides new advantages with each upgrade.

Backed by the long-standing tradition of its publisher John Wiley & Sons, Inc., Thera*Scribe*® comprehensive and flexible nature distinguishes it from other software applications.

► By putting the content of Wiley's best-selling Practice*Planner*® books at the user's fingertips, Thera*Scribe*® provides options for thousands of prewritten clinical management components and tools. This can save hundreds of hours of paperwork and improve the quality of clinical care, while suggesting intervention strategies to the user.

► Thera*Scribe*® is used successfully by providers and practices both large and small.

CHAPTER 1

TheraScribe®

Changes and Enhancements in TheraScribe® 5.0 and Essential 1.0	System Requirements
Activation of TheraScribe®	Installation

Changes and Enhancements in TheraScribe® 5.0 and Essential 1.0

TheraScribe® has a new look, combining many of the powerful tools of previous versions with improved features and important new options.

▶ Easier Navigation

Accessing your information quickly and easily is essential in effectively working with your patients. The new layout of TheraScribe® enables you to do just that. The Navigation Bar is your key to all the TheraScribe® screens and groups of treatment options. The buttons, data grids, and windows within each screen provide clear, direct access to your data.

▶ Changing the Primary Problem/Secondary Problem

You may find it necessary to change your diagnosis of a patient's primary problem while working through his or her treatment plan. TheraScribe® allows you to retain all information gathered and recorded for the initial primary problem while designating it as a secondary problem and choosing a new primary problem area instead.

▶ Editing Lightly and Richly Formatted Reports

TheraScribe® makes editing both lightly and richly formatted reports possible. You can edit any of these reports from within your word processor, using tools that are familiar to you, as you create custom reports that represent your work and practice.

▶ Customizing Screens

You can continue to take advantage of the program's flexibility as you add fields to collect data unique to your own practice, set preferred system defaults, and create custom administrative reports. TheraScribe® also provides powerful new lay-out customization possibilities for all episode-related fields.

▶ Expanded HIPAA Security Settings and Tracking Capabilities

Maintaining HIPAA regulations and security for yourself, your patients, and your practice is increasingly important. TheraScribe® has screens for tracking patient HIPAA information and for regulating settings within the program that are important for maintaining a secure environment.

▶ Timesaving Features

Your search time in the treatment libraries is reduced by displaying only those therapeutic interventions that relate to specific objectives selected for each patient. (The full list of possible interventions can be displayed if desired.) You can create group progress notes in one patient's record and then copy them to other patients who share the same problem and who participated in the same group session. Using the Clinical Pathways set up in TheraScribe® continues to be a valuable part of creating treatment plan and homework plan templates for specific presenting problems.

Expanded Array of Practice*Planners*® Add-On Modules

▶ Previously purchased Treatment Planner modules can be imported into Thera*Scribe*®. In addition, users new to the system, or upgrading users who wish to expand their array of Treatment Planner modules may customize the software to meet their practice needs by purchasing modules for a wide array of specific patient populations (i.e. Addiction, Adolescent Psychotherapy, Family Therapy, Mental Retardation) and treatment settings (i.e. Probation and Parole, College Student Counseling, Early Childhood Education, Rehabilitation, Speech-Language Pathology).

To find a complete listing and to order Treatment Planner modules, visit the Wiley website at www.therascribe.com or call the toll-free Thera*Scribe*® hotline at 1-866-888-5158.

▶ Thera*Scribe*® includes a new set of Progress Notes Planner add-on modules. These modules, which are purchased separately, feature prewritten patient presentation and interventions delivered statements that are tied to the problems, symptoms, and interventions you select for each patient's treatment plan. These time-saving automated and thoroughly integrated progress notes allow users to update treatment records in just minutes.

New Progress Note Planners and add-on modules are constantly being developed. Refer to the Wiley website at www.therascribe.com for a current list.

▶ In addition to Treatment Planner and Progress Notes Planner modules, Thera*Scribe*® supports the use of a number of Homework Planner modules. Designed to correspond with the related Treatment Planner modules, Homework Planners feature exercises designed to engage patients in the treatment process between sessions. Suggestions for assigning and processing the assignments are included in the system. The exercises themselves can be launched as Word files and modified to suit each patient's needs before printing.

Some available Homework Planner modules include: Addiction Treatment, Divorce, Grief, Parenting Skills, and School Counseling. Refer to the Wiley website at www.therascribe.com for a current list.

Website

A hotlink on the Home screen of Thera*Scribe*® links you to the Thera*Scribe*® website

Activation of Thera*Scribe*®

When you are ready to activate:

1. Go to the **Home** screen.
2. Click the red text which reads: **Click here to activate your copy of Thera*Scribe*® 5.0 (or Essential 1.0)**
3. The Activation Wizard will appear.
4. A prompt will ask: Have you purchased a license for Thera*Scribe*®? Click **Yes** or **No**, then **Next**.
5. If you click **Yes**, you will be asked to enter your registration code. (If you are an Essential user, the registration code can be found on the card in the package. If you are a Small Practice or

Enterprise user, the registration code was emailed to you.) If you cannot locate your registration code, please contact your Sales Representative or call 1-866-888-5158.

6. If you click **No,** you will be given information on how to purchase a copy (call 1-866-888-5158 or go to www.therascribe.com)

7. After activation, you will need to restart Thera*Scribe*®. Depending on the edition for which you have registered, you will see the new edition title displayed on the opening screen. If you are running Thera*Scribe*® Essential 1.0, you will enter "**user**" for Username and "**password**" for Password. If you are running Thera*Scribe*® 5.0 Small Practice or Enterprise Editions, you will enter "**admin**" for Username and "**admin**" for Password. For more information about login, refer to the Login section of this manual.

System Requirements

Minimum System Requirements for Installation

COMPONENT	CLIENT PROGRAM	SQL SERVER 2005 EXPRESS
Processor Speed	400 MHz	Minimum: 500 MHz Recommended: 1 GHz or higher
RAM	125 MB	Minimum: 192 MB Recommended: 512 MB or higher
Free Hard Drive Space	100 MB	600 MB
Video Display	SVGA with 256 colors at 800 × 600 resolution	
Operating Software	Windows 2000 or later Internet Explorer 6.0 with Service Pack 1 or later.	Windows Server 2000 SP4 or later, Windows 2000 SP4, Windows XP SP2 or Windows Vista

The database for the Enterprise version can be SQL Server 2000, MSDE 2000, SQL Server 2005, or SQL Server 2005 Express. SQL Server 2005 Express is included on the installation CD.

Installation

Installation Instructions

INITIAL INSTALLATION FOR ALL EDITIONS OF THE THERA*SCRIBE*® 5.0 CLIENT PROGRAM

1. If you wish to install using a CD, insert the Thera*Scribe*® application CD in the CD-ROM drive. If you have downloaded the program, double click to open it.

2. The autorun program should detect the CD and automatically start the Setup program. If it does not, go to **Start, Run,** and enter D:\Setup.exe (where D:\ is the letter for your CD-ROM drive).

3. Click on the **Install** button to install Thera*Scribe*® on the PC. If the install program detects that you do not have all the prerequisites installed, the Thera*Scribe*® Prerequisites Install will be run. Return to step 1 after any reboots. If the prerequisites have are already on the computer, the Thera*Scribe*® install will be run.

4. After the install is complete, launch Thera*Scribe*® from your desktop. A screen will come up asking you to select a database location or to activate your copy of Thera*Scribe*®. If you do not click on the link to activate Thera*Scribe*® and select the database, you will enter **Trial** mode.

5. To enter the Activation Wizard, click on the link to activate Thera*Scribe*®.

> **TIP**
> As with any software installation, it is recommended that you back up your data before installing new software.

6. In the Activation Wizard, click **Next** if you have an Activation Code. Otherwise select **No** and follow the instructions to obtain one. If you selected **Yes** and clicked **Next,** enter your activation code. Your activation code determines which edition of Thera*Scribe*® you will have.

7. Once you enter your activation code, click **Next** and you will have the option to connect over the Internet to activate Thera*Scribe*®, or to contact a Thera*Scribe*® representative. You will be asked to provide the activation code and a machine ID which will be displayed on the wizard.

8. Once you have completed the activation process you will have to restart Thera*Scribe*® to continue.

THERA*SCRIBE*® ESSENTIAL OR TRIAL EDITIONS:
INSTALLATION ON ONE COMPUTER

1. After initial installation, when Thera*Scribe*® Essential is run again you will come to the screen to select a database location. Click on **Create a New Database** button to create a new database.

2. The default login is "**user**" with a password of "**password**".

3. Go to the **Tools Section** and click **Providers.** Click **Password** and change the password to prevent unauthorized access to your data. Record your new password in a secure place so you can easily find it in the event you forget it.

THERA*SCRIBE*® 5.0 SMALL PRACTICE EDITION:
INSTALLATION ON A NETWORK OF UP TO 10 USERS

1. After initial installation, when Thera*Scribe*® is run again you will come to the screen to select a database location. Click on **Create a New**

> **TIP**
>
> The Small Practice Edition uses a Microsoft Access® database. Access® generally performs well in network settings with up to 10 simultaneous users. Customers with more than 10 users and an in-house network administrator should purchase the Enterprise Edition of Thera*Scribe*® 5.0 for optimal system performance.

> **TIP**
>
> To allow applications to share Thera*Scribe*® data, all clients must be mapped to the same directory on the file server where the data file has been copied. All clients must have read/write access to this directory.

Database button to create a new database. Or if one has already been created, you can click on **Open an Existing Data File** to browse for it. If the file is on a network shared drive, the computer must have read/write permissions to that file.

2. If you created a new database, the default login is "**admin**" with a password of "**admin**". Otherwise, if you connected to an existing database, enter the login and password provided to you and skip the remaining steps.

3. Go to the **Tools Section** and click **Providers**. Click **Change Admin Password** and change the admin password to prevent unauthorized access to your data. Record your new password in a secure place so you can easily find it in the event you forget it.

4. If you have activated your copy of Thera*Scribe*® you cannot use the full features of Thera*Scribe*® until you create one or more provider entries on the **Provider** screen and activate them. To do this click **Add** and enter a First and Last Name, and a login name. Also click **Password** to enter a login password. Then click **Activate.** In this process you will have to enter the activation code you used to activate Thera*Scribe*®. Once this is complete you can restart Thera*Scribe*® and login with one of the accounts you created here.

THERA*SCRIBE*® 5.0 ENTERPRISE EDITION: SERVER INSTALLATION

Note: If you have not run the Enterprise Edition Server Installation process or if you do not have an existing SQL Server database then proceed to that first.

If you are using the Enterprise version and do not have a server computer with SQL Server on it, you can use the setup program to install a SQL Server 2005 Express on a computer using the following steps:

1. Insert the Thera*Scribe*® Setup CD in the CD-ROM drive of your server computer.
2. The Autorun program should detect the CD and automatically start the Setup program. If it does not, go to **Start, Run,** and enter D:\AUTORUN.EXE (where D: is the letter for your CD-ROM drive).
3. Click on the **SQL Express** button and go through the setup process. Note: The SQL Server must be configured for Mixed Mode Authentication.
4. Once you have installed SQL Server Express, you need to install and activate Thera*Scribe*® on a client machine using the following steps.

After initial installation, when Thera*Scribe*® is run again, the Thera*Scribe*® login screen will appear. Click on the **Change Connection** button.

1. If a database has not been configured, click on the **Configure** button and go to step 3. Otherwise enter the database server name. If the database name or login account was changed from the default settings in the database configuration process, click the **Database Login** button and enter the login information there. Enter the login and password provided by the person who configured your server and click **OK.** The install process is complete and you can skip the remaining steps.
2. The first screen on the Configuration Wizard gives you the option to create a Thera*Scribe*® database and/or create the login account Thera*Scribe*® uses to connect to the server. When you click **Next,** you will be asked to

enter the server name, a login to the server which has administrator rights and a database name. If you selected the option to create a database, this will be the name of your new database, which cannot be an existing database. If you change the database name from the default value, you will have to set this every time a client machine is configured. If you are just creating the login account, this should refer to an existing Thera*Scribe*® database. Click **Next** to continue.

3. If you selected the option to create a login account, you will be prompted to enter this. These values are set to default values. If you change these values from the default values, every time a client machine is configured, this login information will have to be entered. Click **Next** to continue.

4. Click **Next** on the **Ready to Configure** page to start the process.

5. Once this is complete, you will be brought back to the login screen. Use a login of "**admin**" and a password of "**admin**".

6. Go to the **Tools Section** and click **Providers**. Click **Change Admin Password** and change the admin password to prevent unauthorized access to your data. Record your new password in a secure place so you can easily access it in the event you forget it.

7. If you have activated your copy of Thera*Scribe*®, you cannot use the full features of Thera*Scribe*® until you create one or more provider entries on the **Provider** screen and activate them. To do this click **Add** and enter a First and Last Name, and a login name. Also click **Password** to enter a login password. Then

click **Activate.** In this process you will have to enter the activation code you used to activate Thera*Scribe*®. Once this is complete you can restart Thera*Scribe*® and login with one of the accounts you created here.

IMPORTING PRACTICE*PLANNER*® ADD-ON MODULES

To import data from a new Treatment Planner, Homework Planner, or Progress Notes Planner:

1. Insert the new add-on library CD in your CD drive.
2. Launch the Thera*Scribe*® application from your desktop, and go to the **Database** screen in the **Tools** group.
3. Click the "**Import Planner**" on the screen.
4. Browse for the import file which is located in the Data directory on the CD.
5. The title of the new Practice*Planner*® module will be displayed in the relevant dropdown menus throughout the program.

CHAPTER 2

Feature Overview

Login	Navigation Tool Bars	Working with Clinical Pathways
Home Screen	Types of Fields	Selecting from and Editing Libraries
File Menu	Using Dropdown Lists	Screen Customization
Go Menu	Entering Dates	Exiting the System
Help Menu	Selecting, Adding, and Deleting Patients	

Thera*Scribe*® **uses** a variety of navigational and operational features to help in your use of screens, data entry, selection of patients and Clinical Pathways, use of libraries, and selections through dropdown lists.

Login

The **Login** screen is the central controlling aspect of the security system of Thera*Scribe*®. For confidentiality purposes, Thera*Scribe*® regulates access to patient records. After entering **login name** and **password,** users can select patient records to add or update.

First-time Login for Thera*Scribe*® Trial Edition

Note: The account you create for the Trial Edition is a special account that gives you administrator rights (both full provider and administrator). You can do work using this default user name and password or go to the Provider screen and change your user name and password (see Figure 2.1). You can create provider accounts and work with them without activating each provider.

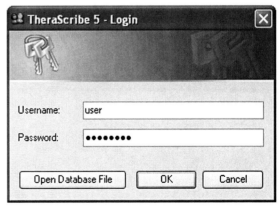

FIGURE 2.1

1. Type "**user**" into the **Username** field of the **Login** window.

2. Type "**password**" into the **Password** field.

3. Click **OK** to gain access to Thera*Scribe*®.

First-time Login for Thera*Scribe*® Essential 1.0

To login, type "**user**" into the **Username** field.

Type "**password**" into the **Password** field.

Click **OK** to gain access to Thera*Scribe*® Essential. You will then be logged on as a single provider and will not need to activate that provider.

First-time Login for Thera*Scribe*® 5.0 Small Practice Edition and Enterprise Edition

Note: The Administrator is able to create and activate provider accounts, but he or she cannot view any patient data and has limited functionality.

1. To login as the Administrator (see Figure 2.2), type "**admin**" into the **Enter Login Name** field.

2. Type "**admin**" as the initial entry password. Click **OK** to gain access to Thera*Scribe*®.

3. Click **Tools Left-Side Navigation Bar** to go to the **Edit Providers** screen.

4. Click **Change Admin Password** at the bottom right of the screen to enter a new secure password for the admin login name.

5. The Administrator should also enter his/her own name and credentials into the provider list by clicking on the name fields and typing in the data. Then click **Security Level** and use the dropdown list to select **Administrator.**

6. Click **Password** to assign a password to the provider who will function as Administrator. This series of steps provides security to the

TIP

It is recommended that you go to the **Provider** screen and change your user name and password for security reasons. The program will warn you to make this change if you have not already done so.

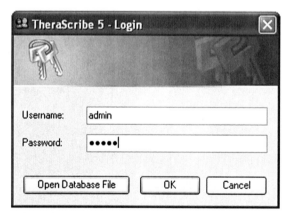

FIGURE 2.2

system as the Administrator tasks will include including adding and deleting providers as well as changing anyone's password.

7. Click **Activate** to work through the activation process for the Administrator.

Assigning Security Levels to Providers

All providers using the system must be assigned their own login name and password by the Administrator. When a provider signs on to the system through the login window, Thera*Scribe*® 5.0 allows that provider to gain access to only those patients to whom he/she has been assigned as Primary Provider, Supervisor, or Team Member. See Tools, Providers for more details.

Home Screen

The **Home** screen will appear whenever you begin work in Thera*Scribe*® (see Figure 2.3). It provides you with easy access to the following key information:

▶ The number of the Thera*Scribe*® version with which you are working

▶ Quick Links (**Add a New Patient, View My Appointment Scheduler, View Sessions**)

▶ Recently selected episodes

▶ Upcoming appointments

▶ Links to other information (Thera*Scribe*® website, E-mail Thera*Scribe*® Technical Support, Download Patient Survey and Other Forms, HIPAA Forms, Suggestion Box, PEC Technologies website)

If you are using the Trial Edition, the **Home** screen provides the Activation link that will enable you to activate full editions of Thera*Scribe*®.

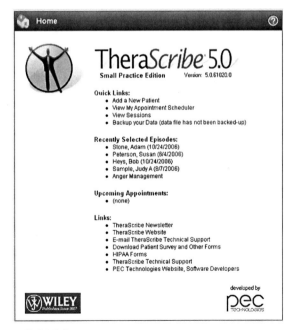

FIGURE 2.3

While working in Thera*Scribe*®, you can return quickly to the **Home** screen by clicking **Home** screen on the Action Bar at the top of the screen.

File Menu

The **File** menu is located on the Menu Bar at the top of your Thera*Scribe*® screen (see Figure 2.4).

▶ It enables you to exit the program.
▶ You can also exit by clicking on the red **X** in the top right corner of your Thera*Scribe*® screen.

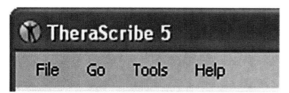

FIGURE 2.4

Go Menu

The **Go** menu is located on the Menu Bar at the top of your screen to give you another way to navigate quickly through Thera*Scribe*® (see Figure 2.5).

▶ You will find ready access to the **Home** screen, **Next** screen, or **Previous** screen with which you were working.
▶ You can also access each of the nine main Navigation Bar screens, with side bars to all group screens.

Help Menu

The **Help** menu is located on the Menu Bar at the top of your Thera*Scribe*® screen.

Using the Help File

1. Click **Help Documentation,** press **F1,** or click the **?** in the top right of the screen to access the Help File related to a particular screen. Thera*Scribe*® includes an extensive screen-related Help File.

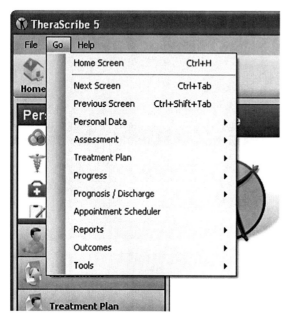

FIGURE 2.5

2. The tabs will allow you to access **Table of Contents, Index, Search,** and **Favorites** for any topic in the program.

Using Other Help Menu Options

▶ Click **Technical Support** for a direct link to the Help File Technical Support information.

▶ Click **TheraScribe Website** to be brought directly to Wiley's Thera*Scribe* website.

▶ Click **About** to view the Thera*Scribe*® splash screen, which indicates the edition you are running (see Figure 2.6).

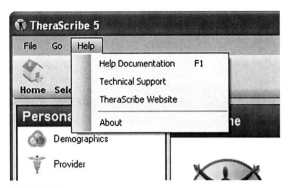

FIGURE 2.6

Navigation Tool Bars

Navigation Bar

Thera*Scribe*® divides the clinical documentation process into several main phases, represented by groups on the Navigation Bar on the left-hand side of the screen (see Figure 2.7):

1. Personal Data
2. Assessment (intake)
3. Treatment Plan
4. Progress
5. Prognosis/Discharge
6. Appointment Scheduler°
7. Reports (print records)
8. Outcomes (data analysis)°
9. Tools

The first several buttons are ordered to reflect a typical clinical process. However, you may choose

°These are not available in the Thera*Scribe*® Essential 1.0 version.

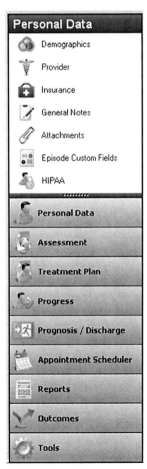

FIGURE 2.7

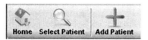

FIGURE 2.8

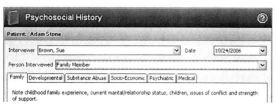

FIGURE 2.9

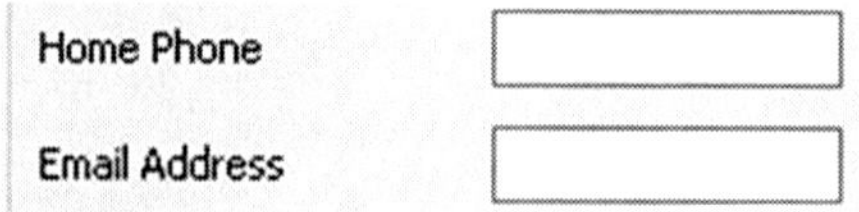

FIGURE 2.10

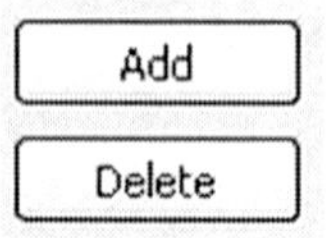

FIGURE 2.11

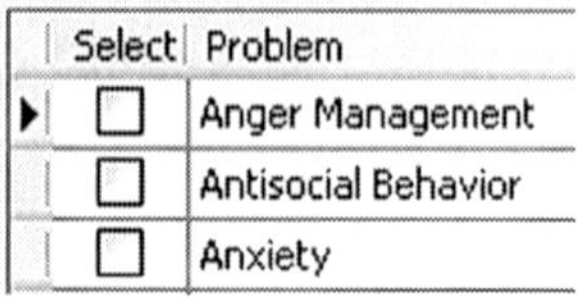

FIGURE 2.12

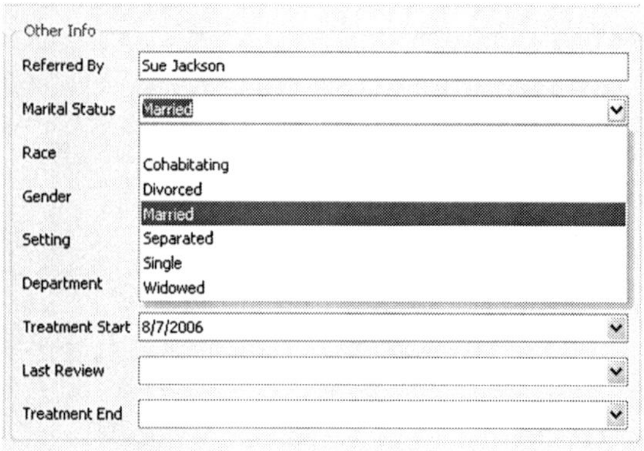

FIGURE 2.13

the areas that best meet your needs, in any order, by clicking the buttons.

Shortcut Bar

Located at the top of the screen, the Shortcut Bar provides quick access to the screens that you use the most (see Figure 2.8). The items in the Shortcut Bar can be customized using the **Tools, Shortcut Bar** screen.

Tab Bars

Two screens in the Assessment Group use a Tab Bar. These are the **Psychosocial History** (see Figure 2.9) and **Mental Status** screens. You can choose between several subsets on each of screen by clicking the appropriate tabs.

Types of Fields

Thera*Scribe*® contains the following types of fields and functions:

- Fields (free-entry text) (see Figure 2.10)
- Buttons (to navigate around program) (see Figure 2.11)
- Check boxes (to select options from long libraries) (see Figure 2.12)
- Dropdown lists (to select from brief libraries) (see Figure 2.13)
- Dropdown calendars (to select dates) (see Figure 2.14)
- Pop-Up Library windows (for extensive libraries) (see Figure 2.15)
- Display fields (where the selections you have chosen from libraries will be displayed) (see Figure 2.16)

▸ Display tables (to enter data in rows) (see Figure 2.17)

Virtually all actions within TheraScribe® can be accomplished with a single click on a field, button, or dropdown list. A click anywhere on a library statement will check the box related to that statement.

Using Blank Fields

TheraScribe® contains a broad array of blank fields, some of which may not be relevant to your practice. You may skip over these fields to leave them blank. However, the field names will appear on the default clinical report. To omit the field names, sophisticated computer users can create custom report formats, using the functions described in the Reports section.

Editing Narrative Fields

TheraScribe® contains a number of narrative fields that allow you to enter an unlimited amount of data for patient history, assessment and treatment summaries, and other text using a rich text format (see Figure 2.18).

You may also use voice recognition software (e.g. Dragon Speak) to dictate into open text fields.

Using Dropdown Lists

TheraScribe® contains a number of dropdown lists (see Figure 2.19). You can click the down arrow to choose from a list of options or make custom selections by typing your own data into the field (except for Provider, Gender, Data Source, and Treatment Phase).

Your customizations will apply only to the current patient record. To make permanent changes to a

TIP
Move between fields by hitting the **Tab** button on the keyboard, or by clicking the mouse cursor on the field.

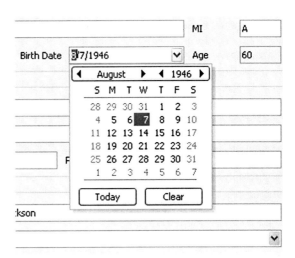

FIGURE 2.14

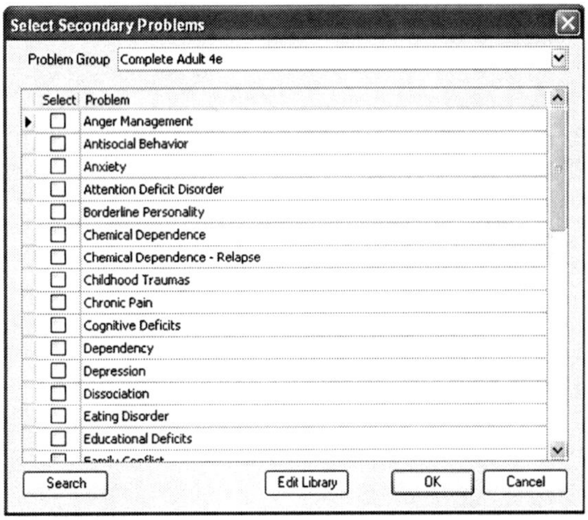

FIGURE 2.15

FIGURE 2.16

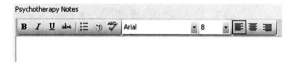

FIGURE 2.17

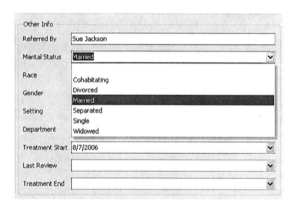

FIGURE 2.18

FIGURE 2.19

TIP

If you wish to select from **All Patients** rather than **Active Patients,** use the dropdown list for the **Select From** field and select **All Patients.** You will then see all patients marked "**Active**" or "**Inactive**" on the **Demographics** screen in the **Personal Data** group.

dropdown list, use the **Libraries** screen in the **Tools** group.

Entering Dates

You can enter dates in TheraScribe® by typing in the date field (i.e. 08/09/1976) or by using the dropdown calendars (see Figure 2.20). To use the dropdown calendars:

1. Click the down arrow to the right of the data field. A calendar will appear.
2. Click **Today** to enter the current date.
3. Click **Clear** to clear the data field.
4. Click on the arrows to the right and left of the month and year to change them.
5. Click the day of the month you wish to enter.

Selecting, Adding, and Deleting Patients

Selecting Patients and Switching Between Patients

To select a patient, click **Select Patient** on the Shortcut Bar near the top of your screen.

▸ You can select an existing patient record by double clicking on the name or by single clicking on the name to highlight it and then pressing the **Select** button (see Figure 2.21). It will default to the latest episode of treatment for all patients in active status unless you change this by clicking the check box for **Show Only Latest Episode.**

▸ Once a patient has been selected, the home screen will appear. Use the Navigation Bar to begin work.

Feature Overview

▶ You can switch between patients from anywhere within the program by clicking **Select Patient** on the Shortcut Bar. You could also click **Home** on the Shortcut Bar and choose a patient from the list of **Recently Selected Episodes.**

Searching for a Specific Patient

You can use the **Search** fields at the bottom of the **Select a Patient** or **Pathway** window to search for a specific patient (see Figure 2.22).

1. Use the dropdown list for **Field** to select what you know about the patient: First Name, Last Name, or ID Number.
2. In the **Value** field, type in the data you choose (e.g., the patient's last name).
3. Any patient records meeting the search criteria you have entered will appear in the data grid above.
4. Select the desired patient.

Viewing Patients by Providers

The **Select a Patient** or **Provider** screen also allows you to view the patients being treated by a specific provider (see Figure 2.23).

1. Use the dropdown list for the **Select From** field and click on **Providers.**
2. Make a Provider selection using the dropdown list for the **Provider** field.
3. Select the patient from the list that appears in the data grid.

Adding Patients

You can add a new patient by doing the following (see Figure 2.24):

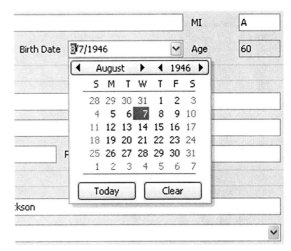

FIGURE 2.20

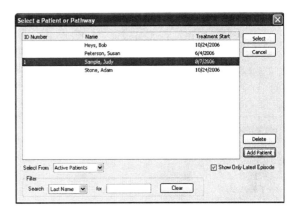

FIGURE 2.21

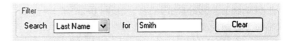

FIGURE 2.22

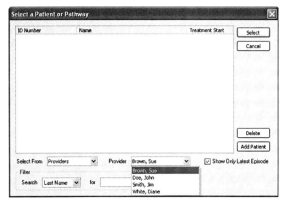

FIGURE 2.23

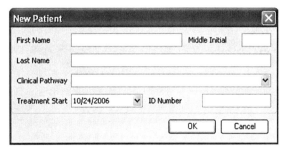

FIGURE 2.24

Instead of deleting a patient, you may want to change the status of the patient to "inactive." To do this, uncheck the **Active** box on the **Demographics** screen in the **Personal Data** group. It is very important, legally, to maintain patient records for several years. Do not consider deleting a record unless you've printed out the complete hard copy report.

1. Click **Add Patient** on the Tool Bar at the top of your screen.
2. A **New Patient** dialog box will allow you to enter the new patient's name, ID number, and treatment start date.
3. If desired, you can also assign a preset Clinical Pathway to the patient.

You can also add new patients while using the **Select a Patient** or **Pathway** screen.

1. Click **Add Patient.**
2. A **New Patient** dialog box will allow you to enter the new patient's name, ID number, and treatment start date.
3. If desired, you can also assign a preset Clinical Pathway to the patient.

Deleting Patients

On the **Select a Patient** or **Pathway** screen, you can also delete a patient, if you have Administrator rights.

1. Select a patient and click **Delete.**
2. A dialog box will ask you if you really want to delete the record, because doing so will permanently delete all the information about that patient.
3. If you click **Yes,** the record will be permanently deleted. Click **No** to return to the **Select a Patient** screen.

Working with Clinical Pathways

Thera*Scribe*® provides you with a powerful tool in its Clinical Pathway function. A Clinical Pathway allows you to designate predetermined problems, definitions, goals, objectives, interventions, and a diagnosis; if desired, it can even include homework assignments for use throughout your time treating a patient. Through insightful use of the Clinical Pathway tool, you can save considerable time in creating treatment plans.

Creating Clinical Pathways

Note: The **Add** and **Edit** Clinical Pathway functions are only available to users with System Administrator security (see Figure 2.25).

1. Log in as a user with Administrator rights.
2. Click **Select Patient** on the Action Bar at the top of your screen.
3. In the **Select a Patient** or **Pathway** window, click on the **Choose From** field and select **Clinical Pathways**.
4. Click **Add Pathway** on the right side of the **Select a Patient** or **Pathway** data grid.
5. A **New Clinical Pathway** window will appear.
6. Enter the name of a new pathway. Click **OK**.
7. Double-click on the new pathway name, or single-click on the pathway name to highlight it, then click **Select**.
8. The **Home** screen will indicate, in red text, that you are working in **Clinical Pathway Mode**. From the **Home** screen, click the **Treatment Plan** button.
9. On the screens in the Treatment Plan section choose the **Problems, Definitions, Goals, Objectives/Interventions, Diagnosis,** and **Homework** you wish to assign to the pathway.
10. In the Homework section, choose the homework assignments you wish to assign to the pathway.

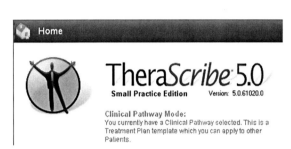

FIGURE 2.25

11. Click the pathway name in the **Name** field at the upper-left corner of the screen to save your selections for the **New Clinical Pathway** and select a patient. The newly created pathway is now available for assignment to any patient.

12. If you click **Delete** when a Clinical Pathway is highlighted on the **Select a Patient** or a **Pathway** window, you will remove that pathway from Thera*Scribe*®.

Editing Clinical Pathway Templates

1. In the **Select Patient** or **Pathway** window, select the **Clinical Pathways** item from the **Choose From** dropdown list (see Figure 2.26). This will display the names of all of the Clinical Pathways that have been created by the Administrator.

2. Select from previously established Clinical Pathways by double-clicking on the desired pathway, or clicking once to highlight the pathway, then clicking **Select.**

3. Click **Treatment Plan** on Navigation Bar.

4. Follow the instructions for the Treatment Plan screens to **add, delete,** or **edit** preselected treatment components.

5. When you are finished, click the **underlined pathway name** in the upper left corner of the screen to select a patient and to save the edited pathway.

Renaming Clinical Pathways

You may decide to rename a Clinical Pathway to better reflect its content or purpose. To do so, simply follow these steps:

1. If you are already working within the pathway, go to **Rename Pathway** screen in the Treatment Plan group.

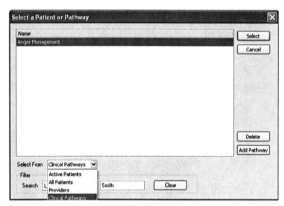

FIGURE 2.26

2. Enter the new name in the dialog box and click **OK.**

3. If you are working with a patient and wish to rename a Clinical Pathway, click **Select Patient** on the Shortcut Bar near the top of your screen and the **Select a Patient** or **Pathway** window will appear.

4. Find the **Select From** field near the bottom of the window and use the dropdown list to select **Clinical Pathways.**

5. Select the **Pathway** you wish to rename from the data grid.

6. On the Navigation Bar, go to the **Rename Pathway** screen in the Treatment Plan group.

7. Enter the new name in the dialog box and click **OK.**

Assigning Preset Clinical Pathways

1. Assign an existing Clinical Pathway to a new patient record by clicking on the **Add Patient** button.

2. Select a preset pathway from the **Clinical Pathway** dropdown list in the **New Patient** window.

3. Once a pathway has been selected, it is applied to the patient. You can customize the treatment plan template for the selected patient by editing within the Treatment Plan section of the program.

4. A Clinical Pathway can also be added to an existing patient's record through the Treatment Plan section on the **Problem** screen.

5. By clicking on the **Assign Clinical Pathway** button, you can assign a pathway to a specific patient.

6. When the selection is complete, Press **OK** to return to the **Problem** screen.

Selecting from and Editing Libraries

Selecting Libraries and Selecting Content

From a wide variety of libraries included in Thera*Scribe*®, you may select and enter statements which you find valuable and informative to include in a patient's clinical record.

There are two types of libraries:

1. General Libraries
2. Practice*Planner*® (Treatment Planner or Progress Note Planner) modules

General Libraries available for your use include:

- Approaches
- Axis IV Stressors
- Complete Axis I Library
- Complete Axis II Library
- Discharge Criteria
- Insurance Carriers
- Medications
- Modality
- Dropdown Lists
- Menus
- Strengths
- Weaknesses

Treatment Planner Libraries include:

- Problems
- Definitions/Symptoms
- Goals
- Objectives/Interventions

- Axis I Diagnosis
- Axis II Diagnosis

Progress Notes Planner Libraries include:

- Presentations
- Interventions

Note: Practice*Planner*® Libraries are only accessible for those add-on modules you have purchased. Call toll-free: 1-866-888-5158 to order Practice*Planner*® Libraries.

To make library selections (see Figure 2.27):

1. Click **Edit Library,** adjacent to each library throughout the program, to display library contents.
2. Click the check box beside the library elements you wish to select for each patient.
3. When you are finished selecting from a library, click **OK.**

Editing Libraries

Users who have been assigned a security level of Advanced or Administrator may edit libraries from within the various sections of the program or from within the Administrator section (see Figure 2.28 and Figure 2.29).

1. Click **Edit Library** in the left-hand corner of the library window.
2. When the library screen pops open, press the **Add** button to the right of the library to add a new entry to the library. For Treatment Planner add-on modules, the program will automatically enter a number to the left of new Definitions, Goals, and Objectives/Interventions.
3. If you **Add** a new **Problem** to a Treatment Planner module, you will need to progress through

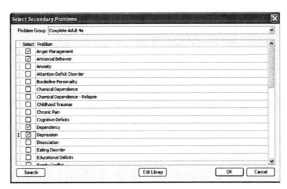

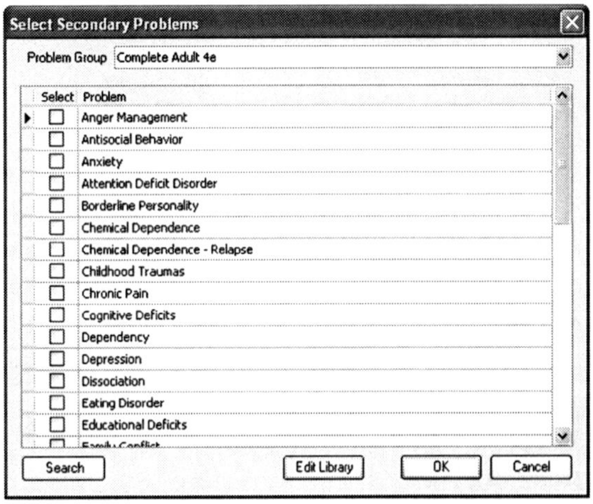

FIGURE 2.27

FIGURE 2.28

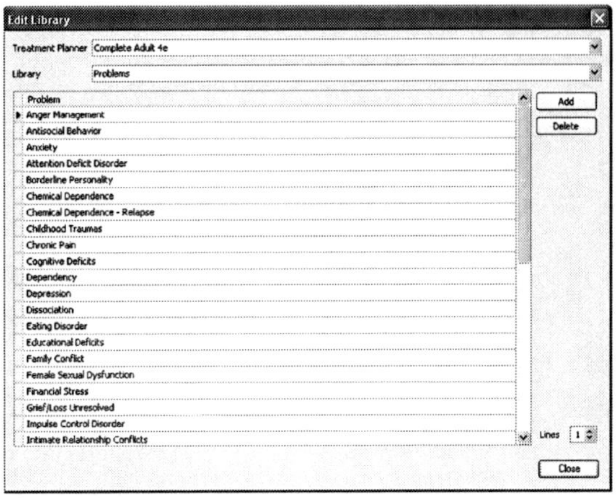

FIGURE 2.29

the Definitions, Goals, Objectives, and Interventions and Diagnosis libraries to add those components to the **Problem.**

4. In addition to adding new content to the libraries, you may **Edit** existing choices within the library by highlighting the item you wish to edit and entering the new text in its place.

5. You may delete any item from the library by clicking on the item to highlight it and then pressing the **Delete** button. Use this function judiciously, as it will permanently remove the item from the database, rendering it unavailable for future patient records.

6. There are links within and between some Treatment Planner and Progress Notes Planner items. To remove built-in content from the add-on modules, you must adhere to the following deletion sequence:

   ▶ Treatment Planner libraries: Deleting a Problem will result in deleting all of the Definitions, Goals, Objectives, Interventions, and Diagnosis associated with that problem.

   ▶ Progress Notes Planner libraries: Deleting any Definitions or Interventions will result in an inability to access the Progress Note Presentation or Progress Note Intervention statements associated with the deleted Definitions or Interventions.

Screen Customization

You are the best determiner of efficient layout, field usage, and key data. The Small Practice and Enterprise editions of Thera*Scribe*® offer powerful new customization capabilities in the area of screen layout for all episode-related fields (see Figure 2.30).

Expand or reduce the number of lines visible for library items by scrolling up or down in the Lines box.

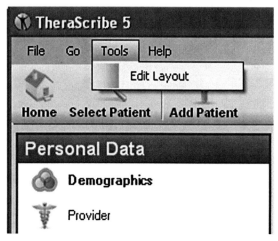

FIGURE 2.30

You have several options for customizing the layout of a particular screen.

Changing the Layout of a Screen

1. Click **Tools** on the Menu Bar at the top of your screen.
2. Click **Edit Layout.**
3. A **Form Layout Customization** window will appear.
4. To rearrange the layout of the screen, click and drag any field to the preferred position. (For example, on the **Demographics** screen, you may want to have **Marital Status** as the first field under **Other Items.** Click on **Marital Status,** which will then highlight in blue, drag it above the **Referred By** field, and drop into place.
5. To see all the items for a particular screen at a glance, click **Layout Tree View.** The highlighted field or section in the **Layout Tree View** will also be highlighted on the gray screen, enabling you to locate the given field or section easily. You can then click and drag to the preferred position.
6. Right click on any field to access the following options (see Figure 2.31):
   ▶ Hide customization form: return to normal screen view
   ▶ Reset Layout: reset screen to original Thera*Scribe*®
   ▶ Rename: type in a different name for the field
   ▶ Hide Text: hide the text for the field, leaving only the data
   ▶ Text Position: use a dropdown list to indicate Top, Bottom, Left, or Right, designating

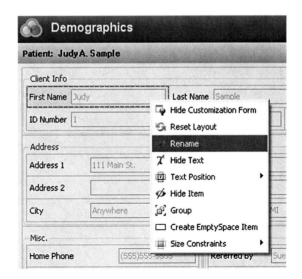

FIGURE 2.31

the position of the text in relationship to the field for the given item

- Hide Item: add the item to the hidden items list for this screen
- Group (if on a group heading): create a new grouping of fields
- Ungroup (in on a group heading): remove the group designation and text heading from the given fields
- Create EmptySpace Item: create an empty space field which can be resized as needed
- Size Constraints: change the size of a given field (Reset to Default, Free Sizing, Lock Size, Lock Width, Lock Height)

Hiding Items on a Screen

1. Click **Tools** on the Menu Bar at the top of your screen.
2. Click **Edit Layout**.
3. A **Form Layout Customization** window will appear (see Figure 2.32).
4. The **Hidden Items** tab will be highlighted, indicating the items that are currently hidden from view on the designated screen.
5. To hide an item, simply click the item on the gray layout and drag it into the **Hidden Items** listing. (For example, on the **Demographics** screen, you may find that you never use the **Military Rank** field. You can easily remove it from the **Demographics Screen** by clicking and dragging it into the **Hidden Items** list.)
6. To hide more items, click and drag.
7. If you want to reset the layout at any time, click **Reset**.

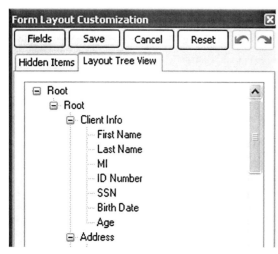

FIGURE 2.32

8. A dialog box will appear, asking you to confirm your desire to set the screen to its original layout.
9. Click **Yes** to reset, **No** to keep your changes.

Using the Fields Button

You can add fields to screens in Thera*Scribe*® by selecting them from any of the episode- or session-related screens or by creating your own custom fields. To add fields:

1. Click **Tools** on the Menu Bar at the top of your screen.
2. Click **Edit Layout.**
3. A **Form Layout Customization** window will appear.
4. Click **Fields** to access the **Layout Fields** window. In this window, you will find a listing of all the session or episode fields included on other Thera*Scribe*® screens.
5. Check the boxes of fields you would like to add to a given screen. Custom Fields can be added to your options here by first going to the **Custom Fields** screen in the **Tools** group and adding them there.
6. Click **OK** to add them to the screen or **Cancel** to return to the screen without making changes.

Saving and Resetting a Screen

1. To save changes to a screen, click **Save.**
2. To cancel changes, click **Cancel.**
3. To reset the screen to its original Thera*Scribe*® layout, click **Reset.**
4. To undo or redo a given change, click the arrows in the top right corner of the **Form Layout Customization** window.

TIP

You can also hide items by right clicking and then clicking **Hide Item.**

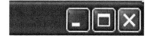

FIGURE 2.33

Exiting the System

The data you have entered will be automatically saved as you move from screen to screen and group to group. When you are done entering data, click the X in the upper-right corner of the screen to Exit the program (see Figure 2.33). Even if you stop midway through creating a treatment plan or making other changes, the data that you entered will be saved.

SECTION II

Application Screens

CHAPTER 3
▶ **Personal Data**

CHAPTER 4
▶ **Assessment**

CHAPTER 5
▶ **Treatment Plan**

CHAPTER 6
▶ **Progress**

CHAPTER 7
▶ **Prognosis/Discharge**

CHAPTER 8
▶ **Appointment Scheduler**

CHAPTER 9
▶ **Reports**

CHAPTER 10
▶ **Outcomes**

CHAPTER 11
▶ **Tools**

Thera*Scribe*® provides nine Navigation Bar groups which allow you to enter and manage all of your clinical documentation.

These include:

- ▶ Personal Data
- ▶ Assessment
- ▶ Treatment Plan
- ▶ Progress
- ▶ Prognosis/Discharge
- ▶ Appointment Scheduler
- ▶ Reports
- ▶ Outcomes
- ▶ Tools

CHAPTER 3

Personal Data

Demographics	Attachments
Provider	Episode Custom Fields
Insurance	HIPAA
General Notes	

The Personal Data group screens help you to manage all the basic information you gather regarding your patient (see Figure 3.1). These areas include demographic data (e.g., birth date, address, phone numbers), provider and insurance coverage information, general clinical notes, file attachments (e.g., spreadsheets, image files), your own custom data fields, and HIPAA-related fields for tracking disclosure authorizations and requested amendments.

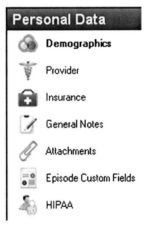

FIGURE 3.1

Demographics

The **Demographic** screen includes the data you entered in the **New Patient** window (Last Name, First Name, Middle Initial, and ID Number). You can edit any of that data here (see Figure 3.2).

▶ You can also enter other information in the appropriate fields: Social Security number, patient's address, phone numbers, employer, and more.

▶ Several dates are represented on the **Demographic** screen. When you enter a **Birth** date, the **Age** of the patient will automatically fill in. The **Treatment Start** date will indicate the date entered in

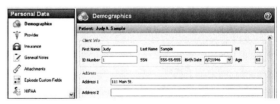

FIGURE 3.2

TIP
Remember, you can leave a field blank if the information does not apply to your work or practice.

the **New Patient** window. To change this date, click the drop-down calendar and select a different date. The **Last Review** field should indicate the most recent date of treatment plan review, and the **Treatment End** field should reflect the date when treatment of the patient ended.

▶ The name you enter for **Psychiatrist** will become the name of the **Prescribing Physician** indicated on the **Approaches** screen in the **Treatment Plan** group. If you do not enter the name of a psychiatrist but do enter a **Primary Care Physician,** the program will default to this name as the **Prescribing Physician** in **Approaches.**

▶ You can indicate if the patient is on Active or Inactive status by clicking the check box for **Is an Active Patient.** Your designation here will determine how his or her name will appear on the **Select a Patient** or a **Pathway** screen. If you choose "**Inactive**," the name will appear only if you select "**All Patients.**"

▶ If this patient has been treated before, click the check box for **This Client was Previously Treated.**

▶ Thera*Scribe*® allows you to maintain records of other Treatment Episodes for a patient treated previously. You can store several independent treatment episodes, complete with dates and treatment plan data, for each patient. If a patient later reenters treatment, simply select the patient's name from the patient list, click **New Episode** on the **Demographics** screen, and proceed with your work. When you enter a new **Start Date** for the patient, the demographic data from previous episodes will automatically copy into the new episode. Previous treatment plan data will not be copied, however, and you can start afresh. Having the option of referring to other Treatment Episodes while focusing on the current needs of your patient will provide valuable insights into treatment approaches.

Provider

The **Provider** screen in the **Personal Data** group displays key information about the primary provider and, if necessary, the supervisor, of treatment for each patient (see Figure 3.3).

Note: This screen does not appear for Thera*Scribe*® Essential version.

▶ You can quickly complete this section for a provider and/or supervisor already entered into the system by clicking the **Name** dropdown list. After you select the appropriate name, other credential information will automatically be displayed.

▶ The Administrator may enter new names and credentials to be included in these dropdown lists by going to the **Providers** screen in the **Tools** group.

▶ You may want to assign a patient to a treatment team or therapy group. Click the **Treatment Team/Group** dropdown list to select the name of the team/group appropriate to the patient's needs.

▶ Assigning a patient to a primary provider, supervisor, or treatment team/group allows all of the providers listed to access and update the patient record. However, only the Administrator may create teams/groups or edit the members of an existing treatment team/group. To do so, use the **Edit Teams/Groups** screen in the **Tools** group.

Insurance

The **Insurance** screen in the **Personal Data** group allows you to select the patient's insurance carrier

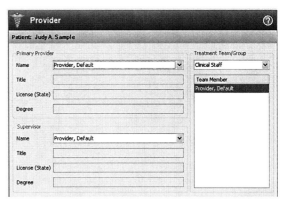

FIGURE 3.3

TIP

Only activated providers can be selected here.

TIP

You can copy progress notes to all patients within a Team/Group. For details on the Progress Notes Copy function see the **Progress, Progress Notes** screen.

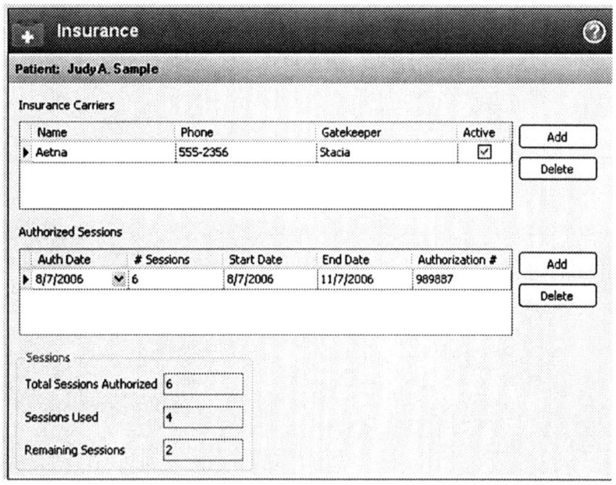

FIGURE 3.4

from the library and apply it to his/her treatment plan (see Figure 3.4). Knowing key insurance information, especially regarding the number of Authorized Sessions and Sessions Used, is very important to the efficient management of your practice.

To select insurance carrier(s), click the **Add** button next to the **Insurance Carriers** data grid. Click on one or more check boxes in the **Select Insurance Carriers** window to select the insurance carrier(s) for the patient, and click **OK.** Enter the **Phone** number and **Gatekeeper** name and click the **Active** check box.

▶ If the patient's insurance carrier is not listed on the checklist, click **Edit Library** in the bottom left corner of the library window to add new insurance carriers to the program. (The **Edit Library** button is visible and available only to users with Advanced or Administrator security levels.)

▶ You can track authorized session information by insurance carrier with the **Authorized Sessions** data grid. First click an insurance carrier name in the top grid and then click **Add** for the **Authorized Sessions** data grid. The **Authorization Date** and **Start Date** fields will default to the current date. You can edit these default dates by using the dropdown calendar. Click in the **#** of **Sessions** to fill in number of sessions authorized, enter the authorization **End Date,** and type in the **authorization #,** if necessary.

▶ You can easily track **Total Sessions Authorized** and **Sessions Used** by looking at the information at the bottom of the **Insurance** screen. As you enter each progress note, the **Sessions Used** tally will increase. Thera*Scribe*® automatically calculates the number of **Remaining Sessions** for you.

TIP

The system Administrator can set warnings on the **Default Setting** screen in the **Tools** group to alert users when the number of authorized sessions is running low or time of authorization is nearing an end date.

General Notes

The **General Notes** screen (see Figure 3.5) in the **Personal Data** group allows you to keep notes to supplement and support clinical information gathered on the other program screens. We recommend that entry of information on this screen be limited to nonsensitive material that can be viewed by a Maintenance level user.

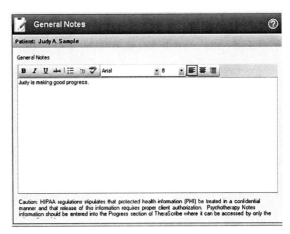

FIGURE 3.5

▶ You can type in an unlimited amount of notes in this rich text field. The tool bar directly above the field enables you to quickly and easily use a variety of word processing functions, including font, point size, color of text, bold text, italics, spell check, underlining, strike through, and justifying text.

▶ If you would like to include these notes in a treatment plan report, include General Notes on the selection list for Clinical Record Reports.

Access to this screen can be kept from Maintenance level users through a check box on the HIPAA screen in the **Tools** section.

Attachments

Different forms of patient information can become important in understanding and treating your patients. Thera*Scribe*® allows you to attach files to a patient's clinical record. These files may include Word files from your patient or other providers. Files may also include scanned documents such as completed psychosocial history forms, children's drawings, or work samples. Image files such as photographs of the patient or other persons in his or her life may also be important to attach.

The **Attachments** screen allows you to attach new files and view or launch previously attached files. If you open a file within Thera*Scribe*®, it will be read-only. If you make changes to the document once it has been opened, save the document under a new name.

Attaching a File

To attach a file to a patient's clinical record (see Figure 3.6):

1. Click **Add** and browse through the directories of the computer to find the name of the file to attach.
2. Click **Open** in the **Open File** window to attach the file. This action will copy the file to the Thera*Scribe*® database.
3. Click **Description** to type in the brief summary of the file attached.

Viewing an Attached File

To view an attached file, click its **Description**. Click **Open File** to view the file as a read-only document.

Editing an Attached File

To edit an attached file, click its **Description**. Click **Open File** to view the file. After editing the file as you desire, click **Save File As** and save it to your hard drive. Reattach the file following the **Add** file process previously described.

Deleting an Attached File

To delete an attached file, click its **Description** of the file that you wish to delete from the Thera*Scribe*® database. Click **Delete**.

Episode Custom Fields

The **Episode Custom Fields** screen (see Figure 3.7) allows you to collect custom data not included

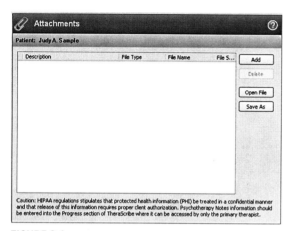

FIGURE 3.6

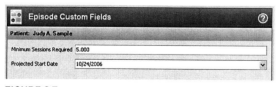

FIGURE 3.7

elsewhere in Thera*Scribe*®. You can take advantage of Thera*Scribe*® flexibility by making customizations for the **Personal Data** group that will capture data unique to your patient base.

The custom fields must be set up by the Administrator in the **Custom Fields** screen in the **Tools** group. Fields may be set up to capture text, dates, currency, and other types of data. The Field Names of the custom fields created by your system administrator are listed in the left-hand side of the screen. Blank data fields to capture the custom data are listed to the right of the custom field name in the Value column.

To enter custom data:

1. Click the **Value** field into which you want to enter data. Click **Edit,** or double-click on the blank value field.
2. A window will open, allowing entry of data through typing on the keyboard or using drop-down lists.
3. Click **OK** when you have finished entering your data.

Advanced users who wish to integrate the fields into appropriate sections of a Clinical Record Report may do so by customizing a report to that end (see Creating Custom Reports in the Reports section).

HIPAA

Maintaining HIPAA standards has become an important part of your work with patients. Thera*Scribe*® offers valuable ways for you to protect your patients and your practice.

The **HIPAA** screen (see Figure 3.8) in the **Personal Data** group provides an easy management tool.

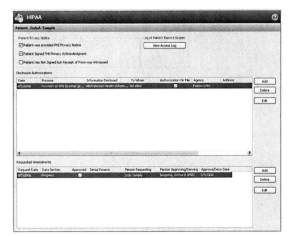

FIGURE 3.8

- Use the check boxes to indicate the status of the Patient Privacy Notice. You can note each of the following, as needed: Patient Was Provided PHI Privacy Notice, Patient Signed PHI Privacy Acknowledgement, and/or Patient Has Not Signed But Receipt of Form Was Witnessed.
- Disclosure Authorizations and Requested Amendments can also be recorded on this HIPAA screen. Click **Add** to the right of either **Disclosure Authorizations** or **Requested Amendments,** and a window will prompt you to fill in the necessary data. Use the dropdown lists when available, or type in custom data. **Edit** and **Delete** are also options for these data grids, if you decide to edit or delete an existing record.
- To view a log of providers who have accessed this patient's record, click **View Log.** Only a user assigned the Administrator level of security and a client's Provider may see the Log of those who have accessed the client's record. The **View Log** will give you data about who opened this patient's record, as well as the date and time that it was accessed. The **Comments** field contains information that indicates that a progress note has been copied into this patient record from another patient's record by a specified provider. The date and time of this copying is displayed as well.

CHAPTER 4

Assessment

Psychosocial History	Mental Status
Strengths/Weaknesses	Recovery
Assessments Given	Summary

The Assessment group screens (see Figure 4.1) are designed to help you record key information as you assess your patient's history, strengths and weaknesses, results of assessments given, and mental status. Thera*Scribe*® gives you clear and manageable structure for this important data as you prepare to make treatment decisions for a patient.

Psychosocial History

The **Psychosocial History** screen (see Figure 4.2) provides an opportunity for you to record narrative summary data in the six areas required by review agencies such as JCAHO, COA, and CARF. Click the tab for each of the following to begin your work:

1. Family
2. Developmental
3. Substance Abuse
4. Socioeconomic
5. Psychiatric
6. Medical

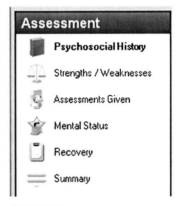

FIGURE 4.1

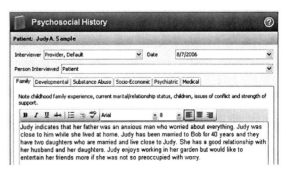

FIGURE 4.2

> **TIP**
>
> Helpful content suggestions are provided for each of these areas along the top of the narrative field. By using these, you will ensure that your text covers the areas required by most agencies and reviewers.

> **TIP**
>
> A Psychosocial History form designed to capture the data needed to compose narrative histories is provided in Microsoft Word® format on Wiley's website. Click on "**Psychosocial History Form**" link on the Home Screen to launch and print the form.

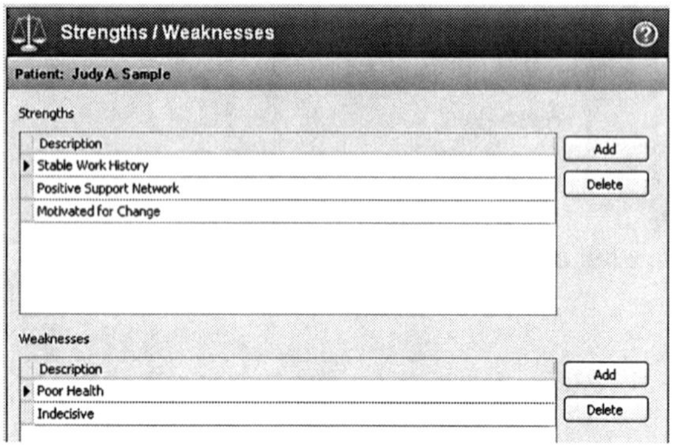

To fill in the other necessary data, which will carry through for all the tab areas:

1. Select the name of the person collecting the psychosocial history data by clicking **Interviewer** dropdown menu and clicking the appropriate name.
2. Record the date that you collected the data by clicking the dropdown calendar.
3. Use the dropdown list to select the **Person Interviewed** (e.g., family member, parent, patient, spouse, teacher).

Strengths/Weaknesses

The **Strengths/Weaknesses** screen in the **Assessment** group provides a selection of words or phrases that allow you to describe a patient's strengths and weaknesses (see Figure 4.3).

▶ By clicking the respective libraries, you can quickly access a comprehensive list to help you in your assessment.

▶ To choose a strength or weakness, click on the check box next to the descriptive words and click **OK** to save your choices. Click **Cancel** to exit the window without saving your selections.

▶ After any item is selected and displayed on the **Strengths/Weaknesses** screen it may be edited for the present patient's treatment plan by clicking on the item. These patient-specific customizations are not saved in the library for use with other patients.

▶ By using TheraScribe® editing capabilities, the Administrator or other users with Advanced security levels can use his or her expertise to make permanent edits or additions to the Strengths and Weaknesses libraries. To do so, click **Edit Library** in the pop-up window and

FIGURE 4.3

make the desired changes. These new or edited choices will then be available for use with all future patients.

Assessments Given

The **Assessments Given** screen in the **Assessments** group (see Figure 4.4) allows you to keep an accurate record of all psychological tests or interviews administered to the patient. Assessments are a fundamental component in forming an effective treatment plan for your patient.

Thera*Scribe*® allows you to select a list of instruments or interviews given, or enter test scores that can be compared in the **Outcomes** group screens.

Selecting an Instrument and Entering Test Scores

1. To select an instrument/interview, click **Add** to the right of the **Instruments** data grid.
2. This will open a **Select Assessment Instruments** window containing interview or test instrument names sorted by **Instrument Group.**
3. There are four types of Instrument Groups built into the Instrument library.
    - Interviews: providing a list of names, no scores (e.g., home evaluation, medication review)
    - Simple Instruments: providing a single score (e.g., Beck Depression Inventory, Trailmaking Test)
    - Other Instrument: providing names, no quantitative results (e.g., Alcohol Use Inventory, Booklet Category Test)
    - Multi-Scale Instruments: providing scores by subscale (MMPI-2® and SCL-90-R®)

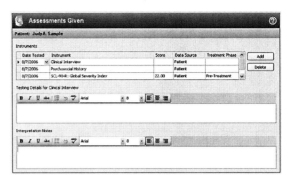

FIGURE 4.4

TIP

Assessment reports and scanned test results or clinical protocols can be attached to the clinical record using the **Attachments** screen in the **Personal Data** group.

> **TIP**
>
> Scores from the Assessment instruments can be graphed in the **Outcomes** group.

4. Click the **Instrument Group** dropdown list to select an instrument category. If you select a multi-scale instrument, a window will provide you with the subscale choices.

5. Check the names of the instruments or subscales that you wish to record for the patient. Click **OK** when you have completed your selection.

6. The names of the instruments or subscales selected will be displayed on the **Assessments Given** screen.

7. Click the **Score** field to enter numerical data that you wish to save in the patient's record.

8. Click the **Data Source** field to select the source of data (system defaults to Patient Self-Report).

9. Click **Treatment Phase** to indicate when instrument was given.

Entering Test-Specific Notes

You may want to enter testing details about specific assessments you administered to your patient. To do this:

1. Click the instrument about which you wish to enter notes.

2. Click the narrative field for **Testing Details** at the bottom of the **Assessments Given** screen.

3. You may enter an unlimited amount of notes in this rich text field.

4. Repeat for other instruments as needed.

Entering General Notes

You may also want to enter notes about the assessment process in general. To do this:

1. Click the narrative field for **Interpretation Notes** at the bottom of the **Assessments Given** screen.

2. Enter an unlimited amount of notes in this rich text field.

Editing the Instrument Library: Basic Instruments

Click **Edit Instruments** at the bottom-left corner of the **Select Assessment Instruments** library window to access the **Assessment Instruments Library** (see Figure 4.5).

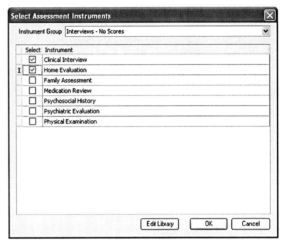

FIGURE 4.5

1. Add **Interviews, Other Instruments,** and **Simple Instruments** by highlighting the type of Instrument you wish to add in the **Instrument Group** box.
2. Click **Add** to the right of the **Interview Type/Instrument** data grid.
3. Click in the **Description** field to type in the name of the interview type or instrument.
4. You may also click in the **Abbreviation** field to type in the initials of the test. This is optional.
5. Click **OK** to add the instrument.

Editing Multi-scale Instruments

To add a **Multi-scale Test** to the **Assessment Instruments Library** click **Add Multi-scale Test** to the right of the **Instrument Group** data grid.

1. Type in the name of the multiscale test in the **Description** field.
2. Click in the **Abbreviation** field to type in a brief name of the test.
3. Click the **Add** button to the right of the **Subscale** data grid.
4. Click in the **Description** field to type in the name of the subscale.
5. Click in the **Abbreviation** field to type in a short name of the subscale.

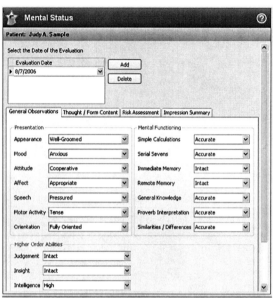

FIGURE 4.6

TIP

As you consider Mental Status in conjunction with your prognosis and discharge criteria, the Navigation Bar allows you to move easily between the **Prognosis/Discharge** screens and **Mental Status** screens.

6. Click **Add** again to type in the name of another subscale and its abbreviation.

7. Repeat this process until all the subscales of the test have been entered. Click **OK.**

Mental Status

The **Mental Status** screen (see Figure 4.6) contains several tabs providing options for making **General Observations,** describing your patient's **Thought Form/Content,** and making a **Risk Assessment** for your patient. Because you may want to make several Mental Status examinations throughout the treatment period, Thera*Scribe*® allows you to enter multiple evaluations. Each evaluation also includes an **Impression Summary** tab.

As you consider your patient's Mental Status, you will be doing so in all three areas each time: General Observations, Thought Form/Content, and Risk Assessment. You will enter data for all three to provide a complete picture, instead of updating data for only one tab.

1. To record a new mental status examination result, click **Add.**

2. If necessary, click on the **Date** field and use the dropdown calendar to change the default date.

Making General Observations

The **General Observation** tab allows you to indicate your overall clinical impression of the patient's mental status using a series of dropdown library lists for three areas:

▶ Presentation (e.g., Appearance, Mood, Attitude, Affect)

▶ Mental Functioning (e.g., Simple Calculations, Serial Sevens, Immediate and Remote Memory)

- Higher Order Abilities (Judgement, Insight, and Intelligence)

To enter General Observations:

1. Click **Add**. The program defaults to descriptors for a well-adjusted, fully functioning person.
2. To change the default descriptors, click the dropdown lists for the fields you wish to change.
3. Because you may have personal observations that differ from the dropdown library lists, you can type in custom descriptors by clicking on any field.
4. Descriptors may be added to or changed for future use on the **Libraries** screen in the **Tools** group.

Describing Thought Form/Content

The **Thought Form/Content** tab offers a quick method of describing the patient's thought form and content through a series of checklists. Three areas of evaluation include:

- Thought Process (e.g., Logical, Illogical, Blocking, Obsessive)
- Delusional Ideation (e.g., None Evident, Persecutory, Grandiosity)
- Hallucinations (e.g., None Evident, Auditory, Visual, Olfactory)

To enter data about your patient's Thought Form/Content:

- Click **Add**. The program defaults to the first check box for normal functioning in these areas.
- If the patient has evidence of pathology in any of the three areas, check the boxes for the applicable pathology-oriented descriptors.

Making a Risk Assessment

The **Risk Assessment** tab allows you to describe the patient's risk of committing Suicide, Violence, Child Abuse, Partner Abuse, or Elder Abuse.

To enter data regarding your patient's Risk Assessment:

1. Click **Add**. The program defaults to no risk for any of these dangerous behaviors.
2. Click on the down arrows to select any increased risk of the patient engaging in these activities, with choices being none, slight, moderate, significant, extreme.
3. Because tracking these behaviors is crucial to monitoring their significance, you can click the **Last Date** field to indicate the last reported incident of the risk behavior. Type in the date or use the dropdown calendar to choose the date.
4. A narrative field with rich text capabilities is available for each risk area so that you can enter any details regarding risk behavior or measures that have been taken to prevent further risk behavior in the future.

Forming an Impression Summary

The **Impression Summary** tab gives you an opportunity to record your overall impressions of the patient's mental status. By using the rich text field to enter an unlimited amount of data, you can provide a valuable summary for quick, future reference as you proceed with your treatment plan.

Recovery

The **Recovery** screen in the **Assessment** group (see Figure 4.7) offers a valuable tool for patient addiction assessment. ASAM has published the Second

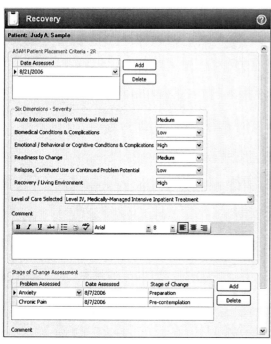

FIGURE 4.7

Edition Revised of its Patient Placement Criteria (ASAM PPC-2R), the most widely used and comprehensive national guidelines for placement, continued stay and discharge of patients with alcohol and other drug problems. With the **Recovery** screen, Thera*Scribe*® allows you to indicate several important things about your patient:

▶ Placement in the Six Dimensions of Severity
▶ Level of Care required with your comments
▶ State of Change Assessment (Problem, Date, and State of Change) with your comments

Make a New Assessment

1. Click **Add** to begin recording a new Recovery Assessment.
2. The date will default to the current date; use the dropdown calendar to change the date.
3. You can rate each of the Six Dimensions of Severity by clicking the dropdown list and selecting **Low, Medium,** or **High.**
4. Use the dropdown list to select a **Level of Care** (Early Intervention, Outpatient Treatment, Intensive Outpatient/Partial Hospitalization, Residential/Inpatient Treatment, Medically Managed Intensive Inpatient Treatment)
5. The rich text **Comments** field allows you to make narrative observations about your assessment.

Making a State of Change Assessment

1. Click **Add.**
2. Enter **Problem Assessed, Date Assessed,** and **State of Change** using the dropdown lists.
3. Use the rich text **Comments** field to make narrative observations.

Summary

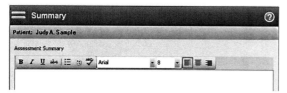

FIGURE 4.8

The **Summary** screen provides the option for entering a narrative summary of unlimited length in rich text format, describing the assessment process and related information as a whole (see Figure 4.8). You may choose to leave the field blank or to enter an overall testing report or summary of results.

CHAPTER 5

Treatment Plan

Problem	Objectives/Interventions	Diagnosis
Definitions	Modality	Response
Goals	Approach	Homework

The Treatment Plan screens (see Figure 5.1) provide a master framework designed to guide you through the process of creating an effective treatment plan for your patient. Arranged sequentially, as you will probably approach your work, each screen addresses a specific component of the treatment plan. These include:

1. Problem
2. Definitions
3. Goals
4. Objectives/Interventions
5. Modality
6. Approach
7. Diagnosis
8. Response
9. Homework

The Thera*Scribe*® add-on module libraries provide you with a wide array of important options, depending on patient needs. To use the Treatment Plan components, you will need to install at least one of the many Treatment Planner modules available.

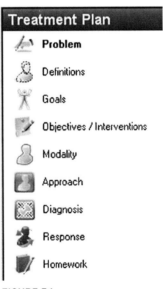

FIGURE 5.1

TIP

In order to add new treatment plan elements to a specific patient, users with Basic level security will need to select a treatment plan component they do not wish to use, then type over the undesired component in the display box. Users with Advanced or Administrator level security can also use the type-over method to make additions to a specific patient's treatment plan, or they may make permanent changes or additions to the **Treatment Plan** libraries by using the **Libraries** screen in the **Tools** or by using the **Edit Libraries** button.

Adding to or Editing Treatment Plan Libraries

All of the **Treatment Plan** screens have identical processes for adding, editing, and deleting selections from libraries.

Once you have selected statements from the **Treatment Plan** libraries, Thera*Scribe*® gives you the flexibility of editing them for the specific patient record by clicking on the statement in the display window and then typing in your changes of text.

Using Clinical Pathways

In the course of your work, you may often find that you are treating patients with similar presenting problems. If this is true, Clinical Pathways may be of definite interest to you. By using a Clinical Pathway, you can assign problem templates with your preferred Definitions, Goals, Objectives, Interventions, Diagnoses, and Homework to use time after time.

As you work with individual patients, you can use the Clinical Pathway as a basic treatment plan and fine-tune it to meet varying needs.

To bring treatment plan data in a Clinical Pathway over to your patient, click the **Assign Clinical Pathway** button on the **Problem** screen.

Problem

The **Problem** screen in the **Treatment Plan** group allows you to designate presenting problems for the patient (see Figure 5.2).

You may commonly make a dual diagnosis. However, most third-party payors require a primary DSM-IV® code for remittance. Therefore, a **Primary** problem must be designated.

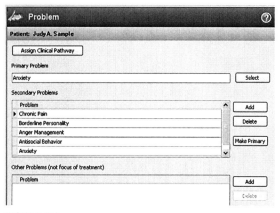

FIGURE 5.2

Treatment Plan

Secondary problems are other problems of importance that will be addressed in the treatment plan.

The **Other** category may be used to note problems that have been discovered through the psychosocial assessment but will not be addressed in treatment at this time.

Selecting Problems from Treatment Planner Libraries

As you identify the patient's problems, the **Treatment Planner** libraries become very useful, providing comprehensive lists for many categories of presenting problems.

1. To choose a **Primary Problem,** click the **Select** button to bring up the **Select Problem** window, displaying a list of problems.

2. Click the **Problem Group** down arrow to display a dropdown list of treatment planner library modules that have been purchased and imported into Thera*Scribe*®.

3. Click on the **Treatment Planner Library** module (e.g., Adult, Adolescent, Addiction) that is appropriate for the current patient.

4. From the list of problems available in the chosen treatment planner module, check the **Primary Problem** and Click **OK** (only one **Primary Problem** may be selected).

5. To select one or more secondary problems, click the **Add** button to the right of the **Secondary Problems** field. The same library of problems will again be displayed, and you may check one or more secondary problems. Click an item again to unselect it. When you are satisfied with your choices, click **OK**.

Each of us works differently. Continue to design the Treatment Plan in a sequence that best works for you. After you have selected presenting problems from the **Problem** screen, you may proceed through the other screens (e.g., **Definitions, Goals, Objectives/Interventions**), one by one for the problem selected. That problem will automatically remain at the top of your screen for ease of use until you use the dropdown list again to select a different problem.

Or, you can focus on each step of the Treatment Plan itself, first finding **Definitions** for each **Problem**, then setting **Goals** for each problem, and so on. To take this approach, simply use the dropdown list to switch between problems as you work.

TIP

Thera*Scribe*® provides you with a notable new option on the Problem screen. If you decide to change your primary diagnoses during the course of your work with a patient, the current Primary Problem will be included in the Secondary Problem list. If you decide to make a designated Secondary Problem the Primary Problem, you can simply click **Make Primary** and the old Primary Problem will automatically switch to the **Secondary Problem** field. In either case, all data will be saved.

6. To select **Other Problems,** click the **Add** button. Use this field to acknowledge problems you see in the patient that you will not be specifically addressing in the current treatment plan. Click **OK** to continue.

7. Click **Definitions** on the left-side Navigation Bar to proceed to the next section, which will provide behavioral definitions for each of the problems you have designated.

Selecting a New Primary Problem

You may also want to select a new problem to designate as **Primary** by doing the following:

1. Add the problem to the **Secondary Problem** list.
2. Then click on **Make Primary** to move it to the **Primary Problem** field. The former Primary Problem will simultaneously move to the Secondary Problem list, with its associated data saved.

Definitions

The **Definitions** screen (see Figure 5.3) provides meaning and clarity as it allows you to describe the problems selected in the Problems screen. Because individual patients present problems in different ways, you need the flexibility of a wide array of descriptions that the Thera*Scribe*® libraries provide.

1. Click the dropdown list to see the list of problems you have decided to focus on with your patient.
2. Click the problem you wish to define.
3. When you click **Add,** a **Behavioral Definitions** library window will appear, with a list of behavioral definitions for the target problem.

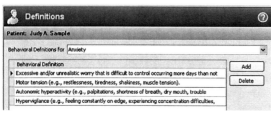

FIGURE 5.3

4. By using the up and down arrows by the **Lines** field, you can increase or decrease the amount of lines available for each definition.

5. Click the items you would like to select from the library. Click an item again to unselect it.

6. When you are finished, click **OK** at the bottom of the window.

7. At this point, you can continue by selecting another problem from the dropdown list. Or, you can click **Objectives/Interventions** in the **Treatment Plan** group on the left-side Navigation Bar to proceed to the next section of the plan.

Goals

The **Goals** screen allows you to set goals for your patient, having identified and defined his or her problem areas (see Figure 5.4).

1. Click the dropdown list to see the list of problems you have decided to focus on with your patient.

2. Select the problem for which you intend to set some goals.

3. When you click **Add,** a **Goals** library window will appear, with a list of goals for the target problem.

4. By using the up and down arrows by the **Lines** field, you can increase or decrease the amount of lines available for each goal description.

5. Click the items you would like to select from the library. Click an item again to unselect it.

6. When you are finished, click **OK** at the bottom of the window.

7. At this point, you can continue by selecting another problem from the dropdown list. Or,

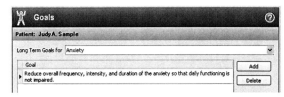

FIGURE 5.4

you can click **Goals in the Treatment Plan** group on the left-side Navigation Bar to proceed to the next section of your plan.

Objectives/Interventions

To reach their treatment goals, your patients must take smaller steps toward achieving the good. You need to ask: "What do I want this patient to do?" These actions are called Objectives. Objectives are expressed in behaviorally specific terms, identifying behaviors which can be observed and, whenever possible, quantified or measured.

You, then, will try to enable your patient to achieve the objectives with a variety of Interventions.

Note: Newer Planner modules will include Evidence-Based Treatment (EBT) designations for some objectives.

Selecting Objectives for Problems

You will use the following steps to select **Objectives** from the **Objectives/Interventions** screen libraries (see Figure 5.5).

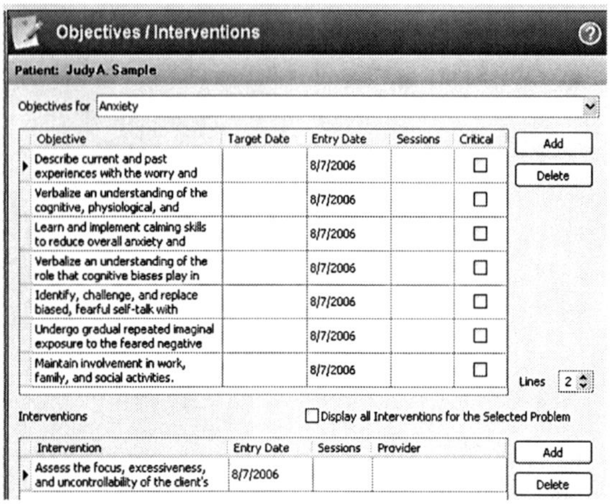

1. Click the dropdown list to see the list of problems you have decided to focus on with your patient.
2. Select the problem for which you intend to determine Objectives.
3. When you click **Add** to the right of the **Objective** data grid, a **Select Objective** library window will appear, with a list of objectives for that specific problem.
4. By using the up and down arrows by the Lines field, you can increase or decrease the amount of lines available for each Objective description.

FIGURE 5.5

5. Click the check boxes by the items you would like to select from the library. Click an item again to unselect it.

6. When you are finished, click **OK** at the bottom of the window.

7. You can also enter the **Target Date** (for achieving the objective), the **Entry Date** (at which the patient began treatment), and **Sessions** (predicted necessary to achieve the objective). By clicking the check box for **Critical,** you are indicating that a given objective is critical to the discharge of the patient from treatment.

8. At this point, you can continue by selecting another problem from the dropdown list and repeating steps 3–7. Or, you can move to the **Interventions** section of the screen.

Selecting Interventions for Objectives

As you consider what interventions to use for achieving each objective, Thera*Scribe*® can provide valuable help. It links objectives with the interventions most likely to help the patient achieve those objectives. You can create these important links by following these steps:

1. In the display field at the top of the screen showing the objectives you selected, click and highlight an objective for which you wish to select interventions.

2. Click the **Add** button beside the **Interventions** display field on the bottom half of the screen.

3. A selection of the interventions most commonly used for the highlighted objective will appear in a library window.

4. The interventions that appear are those most likely to be used to treat the highlighted objective. To select from this short list, click the

> **TIP**
>
> The data in the **Objectives/Interventions** screen defaults to show only the interventions selected for the highlighted objective. To view all of the interventions selected for a patient, check the **Display all Interventions for Selected Problem** box on the main **Objectives/Intervention** screen.

check boxes for the interventions you wish to use, and click **OK**.

5. The interventions shown are part of a more extensive list of possible interventions for the problem. If you wish to choose from all of the possible interventions for the target problem, click the check box for **Show All Interventions for this Problem** at the bottom of the library window.

6. When you are finished selecting interventions for the highlighted objective, click **OK**.

7. The **Entry Date** will default to the current date. To change the date, use the dropdown calendar.

8. You have the option to enter number of sessions during which the intervention will be implemented in the **Sessions** column of the **Interventions** data grid. You then use the down arrow to select the provider responsible for delivery of the intervention. (It will default to the provider who is logged on.)

9. Click on the next objective at the top of the tab screen, and repeat steps 2 through 8.

Modality

The **Modality** screen is used to specify the treatment modalities and frequency of each type of therapeutic contact (see Figure 5.6). Some of the choices for modalities are general, such as **Individual or Family Therapy, Group Therapy, Occupational Psychotherapy,** or **Medication Management Psychotherapy.** Other choices are more specific and tied to CPT codes.

You can also designate the level of care that will be used and make general narrative notes regarding each modality.

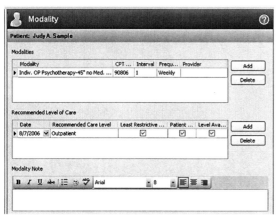

FIGURE 5.6

Selecting Modalities

To select modalities:

1. Click **Add** to the right of the **Modality** grid. A **Select Modalities** window will appear.

2. Click the check boxes for the modalities you wish to choose.

3. Click or use the tab button on your keyboard to move through and complete the **Frequency, Interval,** and responsible **Provider** fields for each selected modality, using dropdown lists to help you. The CPT code will fill in automatically if it was specifically designated in the library.

Selecting Recommended Level of Care

As the level of care for a patient may change throughout the treatment episode, Thera*Scribe*® allows you to recommend different levels of care by date.

1. To enter a level of care, click Add to the right of the **Recommended Level of Care** data grid.

2. A new row will appear, defaulting to the current date. Select a different date, if needed, by using the dropdown calendar.

3. Select a recommended care level from the dropdown list or type in a custom level of care.

4. Three check boxes in this data grid allow you to give more information about the selected **Level of Care.** These are: **Least Restrictive Alternative, Patient Agrees** (with level of care assignment), and **Level Available.** They will default to the "on" status. If necessary, you may change them by clicking on the check box.

Entering Modality Notes

The **Modality Note** narrative field at the bottom of the **Modality** screen allows you to type in a general narrative note in rich text format. You can elaborate on the details of any or all of the treatment modalities that have been selected.

For example, you describe the topic and purpose of a focus group, note the times and dates that specific group will be held, or provide reasons for the designated level of care or changes in that care.

Approach

The **Approach** screen in the **Treatment Plan** group allows you to choose therapeutic approaches that you will take with your patient (see Figure 5.7).

Options given include: Behavioral Techniques, Biofeedback/Relaxation Training, Cognitive Restructuring, Confrontive, Insight Oriented, Solution Oriented, Supportive Maintenance, and Symptom Focused Education.

If medications are prescribed, dosages, frequency, and other medication details may be tracked on the Approach screen, since these may play a key role in your approach to treating your patient.

Selecting Treatment Approaches

To select an **Approach:**

1. Click **Add** to the right of the **Approaches** data grid.
2. The **Select Treatment Approaches** library window will appear.
3. Click one or more check boxes to select desired treatment approaches. Click **OK.**

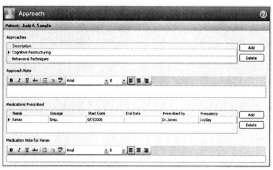

FIGURE 5.7

4. You may enter comments and observations about the various approaches and their impact on your patient by using the **Approach Note** narrative field. Rich text format is available.

Selecting Medications

To add new Medications Prescribed by the primary clinician or a treating physician:

1. Click **Add** to the right of the **Medications Prescribed** data grid.
2. The **Select Medications** window will show the medications listed in the Medication Library.
3. Medications are sorted by class, as follows: **Anti-ADD/ADHDs, Anti-Anxieties, Anti-Depressants, Anti-Parkinsonians, Anti-Psychotics, Hypnotics/Sedatives,** and **Mood Stabilizers.** Use the drop-down list to select a general class of medication.
4. Click on the check box to select a specific medication or medications from within the general classes.
5. Click **OK** to display the medications in the data grid on the **Approaches** screen.
6. Click the **Start Date, End Date, Dosage, Frequency,** and **Prescribed by** to the right of each medication name to enter these details.

TIP

The **Prescribed by** field will default to the name the Psychiatrist entered on the **Demographics** screen. If no Psychiatrist is listed, it will default to the Primary Care Physician. Defaults can be overridden by typing in a new name.

Entering Medication Response Notes

Narrative details regarding your patient's response to each medication can be typed under Notes for Medications, using a rich text format.

1. Click the medication you wish to describe in the **Medications Prescribed** list to highlight it.
2. Enter comments about the patient's response to that specific medication in the **Medications Note** narrative field.

3. Click a different medication in the **Medications Prescribed** box to open a new narrative field for each medication.

Diagnosis

The Diagnosis screen (see Figure 5.8) allows you to assign DSM® or ICD-9® diagnoses for your patient.

Based upon the Primary Problem selected in the Problem screen, Thera*Scribe*® suggests Axis I (clinical disorders) and Axis II (personality disorders and mental retardation) diagnoses for your consideration.

Moving beyond these diagnoses, you can also to enter or select:

▶ Axis III physical problems (Medical conditions that impact care)

▶ Axis IV stressors (e.g., Economic, Family Conflict, Education Deficit)

▶ Axis V Functioning Levels (GAF score based on a scale of 1–100)

▶ Stress Severity Ratings (None, Mild, Moderate, Severe, or Extreme)

1. Click **Add** next to the **Axis I Diagnosis** data grid. The **Select Axis I Diagnoses** library window will appear.
2. If the diagnosis appropriate for your patient is not displayed, click the check box labeled **Show Complete Axis I Library.** You may click the dropdown list to select ICD-9 diagnoses.
3. Click one or more the check boxes for the appropriate diagnosis/diagnoses for your patient.
4. Click **OK** to display the selected diagnosis/diagnoses.

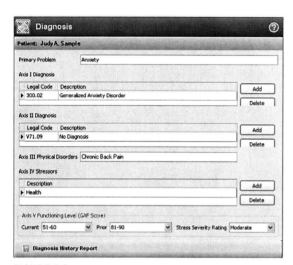

FIGURE 5.8

5. Repeat steps 1 through 4 for the **Axis II** data grid.

6. Click the **Axis III Physical Disorders** field to type in any medical conditions that impact the patient's mental or emotional well-being.

7. Enter **Axis IV Stressors** by clicking **Add** next to the **Stressors** data grid. Check all appropriate stressors, and click **OK.**

8. Current and Prior **Axis V Functioning Levels** can be entered by using the appropriate dropdown lists and clicking the rating of your choice. Monitoring current and prior GAF scores will help you to evaluate your patient's status and may provide needed data for insurance and Social Security records. These ratings may be deleted and left blank if the user wants to change to no rating at a later time.

9. Descriptive Stress Severity Ratings may be selected in the **Stress Severity** box.

Response

The **Response** screen provides two rich text narrative fields for recording your assessment of responses to the Treatment Plan (see Figure 5.9). Click in either field to type.

▶ In the **Patient Response** field, you can keep anecdotal records of your patient's input and reactions to his or her treatment plan, with your comments when appropriate.

▶ In the **Significant Other's Response** field, you describe the reaction of others, like a spouse, partner, parent, guardian, or mentor of your patient. Because the significant other interacts with your patient in intimate and unique ways, recording his or her reactions to the treatment

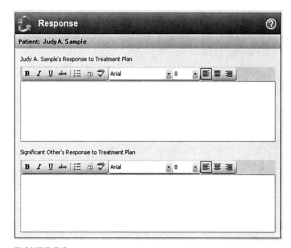

FIGURE 5.9

plan and its impact on your patient may provide valuable insights to help you in your work.

Homework

The **Homework** screen provides invaluable help to you as the clinician. You want to keep your patients engaged in the treatment process between sessions. To do so, you need to provide concrete activities that give guidance in meeting objectives and require accountability to the treatment process.

Thera*Scribe*® offers a set of Homework Planner add-on modules. The Homework Planners consist of prewritten exercises that give you the ability to plan effective homework and stimulating guides for discussion with the click of the mouse.

Homework libraries are available for the following patient groups:

- Adult (two available)
- Adolescent (two available)
- Child
- Chemical Dependence / Addiction
- Couples
- Divorce (relates to couples treatment)
- Employee Assistance
- Family
- Grief (relates to adult treatment)
- Group Therapy
- Parenting Skills
- School Counseling

Homework assignments are treated as interventions. Therefore, Thera*Scribe*® automatically links the specific problems and objectives you identified for your patient on the other Treatment Planner screens to the options offered by the Homework Planner libraries.

Note: Additional Homework libraries may become available periodically.

Selecting Homework Assignments

1. The problems selected for the patient on the **Problem** screen are displayed in the **Homework for** dropdown list at the top of the **Homework** screen (see Figure 5.10).

2. Click the down arrow to display all of the problems previously selected, and choose one of them for which you wish to assign homework.

3. The **Objectives** that have been previously selected for that problem will be displayed.

4. Select any one of the objectives for association with a particular homework assignment by clicking on the objective.

5. Once an objective is selected, Click **Add** to the right of the **Homework** data grid. The **Select Homework** library window will appear.

6. The **Select Homework** library will default to display the homework titles for the problem focus. The dropdown list also allows you to select the entire listing of homework titles from the Homework Planner associated with the Treatment Planner you are using for this patient. Note: If no selections appear in the window, use the dropdown list to select the entire listing.

7. Considering the particular objective you have in mind, click the check boxes to select the titles of homework that you think will best help your patient meet the objective. To assist you in your selection, the goals for each assignment will appear when the cursor rolls over the title

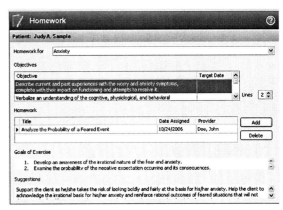

FIGURE 5.10

> **TIP**
>
> In the Homework Assignment library window, assignments most closely tied to the problem you selected on the main **Homework** screen are indicated as **Primary**. Additional assignments from the **Homework Planner** module are also listed, but not as **Primary**.

of the assignment. More than one homework assignment may be selected. Click **OK** when you have completed your selections.

8. The titles of the homework assignments you selected will be listed as interventions delivered for the related objective in the patient's Clinical Record report.

9. After you select an exercise, Thera*Scribe*® provides more helpful information at the bottom of the screen. The **Goals of Exercise** field lists several goals that this homework assignment may help your patient to achieve. Having these clearly described enables you to assess the appropriateness of the given assignment and allows you to present the homework in the most effective way. The **Suggestions** field provides several questions that can help your patient to process the homework, both at the time it is assigned and after it has been completed.

10. If Microsoft Word® is installed on your computer, you may view a homework assignment on the screen by clicking **Launch** to the right of the **Homework** data grid. The homework assignment will be displayed on the screen. It can be edited, if necessary. Then you can print it and send it home with your patient.

11. Repeat steps 2 through 10 to assign homework for other problems and objectives.

CHAPTER 6
Progress

- Session Details
- Progress Notes Planner
- Objective Rating
- Psychotherapy Notes
- Session Custom Fields
- Amendments

The **Progress group screens** help you to monitor a key component in your patient's treatment plan: progress (see Figure 6.1). Thera*Scribe*® provides a data grid to display Session Details, a Progress Notes Planner to enter notes, an **Objective Rating** screen to track objectives, and two other areas to track **Psychotherapy Notes** and **Amendments to the Progress Notes.**

Using the Locking Feature for Progress Notes

A locking feature is available to provide security and privacy for your patients (see Figure 6.2). To enable or disable this feature, go to the **System Settings** screen in the **Tools** group.

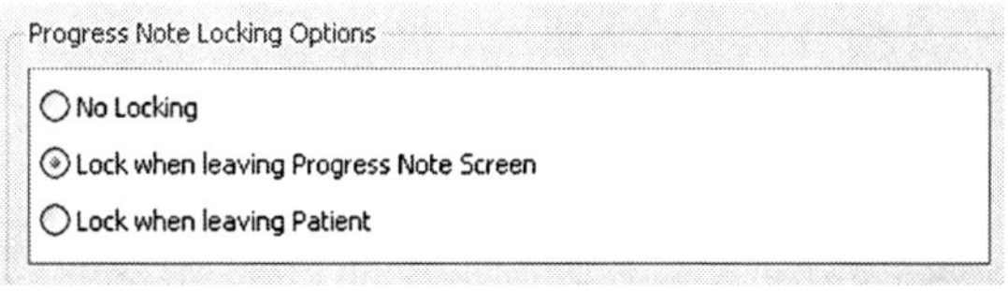

Note: Be advised! Depending of your choice of locking feature, when you leave the screen or the patient you will lock the data and will not be allowed to change it. You will need to make an amendment.

If the progress note locking feature is enabled:

▶ The **Lock Date** field will fill automatically with the date that a progress note is created. If they are locked, notes cannot be edited or deleted after they are initially entered.

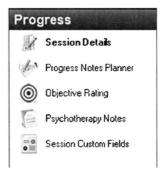

FIGURE 6.1

FIGURE 6.2

TIP

You may choose between three versions of the locking feature:

▶ Lock when leaving **Progress Notes** screen.
▶ Lock when leaving patient file selected.
▶ No Locking.

- To make changes to a note, you will need to use the **Amendments** screen in the **Progress** group. This will allow you to add a change to a progress note. This change, or amendment, will also be locked and dated.
- The **Session Details** data grid is visible to all providers who have security access to the patient's record.
- The progress note data (**Progress Notes Planner, Objective Rating, Psychotherapy Notes,** and **Amendments**) on the bottom half of the screen is only visible to the patient's Primary Provider and the Team Member who created a progress note. The Team Member can only see a note that he or she has created, while the Primary Provider can see all progress notes. This feature can be enabled or disabled within the **Tools** group of the program on the **System Settings** screen.

Session Details

The **Session Details** screen in the **Progress** group provides a clear overview of the time you have spent with the patient (see Figure 6.3). The data grid appearing at the top of this screen will appear for your reference at the top of each of the screens in the **Progress** group. Information on the **Session Details** screen includes:

- Date of the session
- Start and End times
- Length of session
- A check box to indicate whether the session was Billable
- Session Number (Note: A session will not be counted in the session number field if it is not checked as billable.)

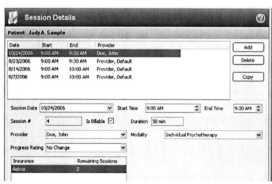

FIGURE 6.3

- Provider
- Modality used
- Progress Rating
- Insurance information

Entering Session Details

Contacts are sorted in inverted order, with the most recent session listed at the top of the **Session Details** field. This allows you to access your most recent data quickly and easily.

To enter a session:

1. Click **Add** to the right of the **Session Details** data grid.
2. Thera*Scribe*® will automatically enter a new Session Number and the current date into the **Date** field. If necessary, the default date can be changed by using the dropdown calendar.
3. Enter the **Start time** and **End time** in the appropriate boxes. Start and End times for subsequent contacts will default to those times that were used for the previous entry. If necessary, the default times can be altered by clicking on the fields.
4. Based upon the times entered in the **Start** and **End** fields, the **Length** of the session will be automatically calculated.
5. The **Billable** contact field will default to the "on" position. Contacts which won't be charged (e.g., phone contact) must be unchecked. Otherwise, they will be subtracted from the number of authorized sessions remaining.
6. The **Provider** field will default to the current user's name. You can override this default by

clicking in the field and choosing a different provider from the dropdown list.

7. Select a **Modality** from the dropdown menu. Once a **Modality** is selected, future sessions will default to that modality unless you choose to select a different one.

8. The **Progress Rating** field will default to "**Some Progress.**" You can make a different selection (**Significant Regression, Regression, No Change,** or **Completed**) by clicking on the field and choosing from the dropdown list.

9. If the **Progress Note** locking feature is enabled, the **Lock Date** field will fill automatically with the date that a **Progress Note** is created and locked into the database.

10. Use the dropdown list to enter the name of the **Insurance** into the data grid.

11. Based upon whether the contact is marked as Billable, Thera*Scribe*® will calculate **Authorized Sessions Remaining.** This is based on the number of authorized sessions entered in the **Insurance** tab of the **Personal Data.**

The system administrator may establish when this warning appears. To do so, he or she can make selections on the **Default Settings** screen in the **Tools** group, based on number of sessions or days remaining.

Progress Notes Planner

The **Progress Notes** screen gives you the opportunity to record progress notes, both prewritten and narrative (see Figure 6.4).

The prewritten notes are possible through the use of Thera*Scribe*® add-on Progress Notes Planner libraries, which correspond to the Treatment Planners of the same name.

As you approach the limit on the number of authorized sessions or date range, a warning message will be displayed on the **Progress** screen reminding you to check authorization parameters. The warning message also appears when the patient's name is selected.

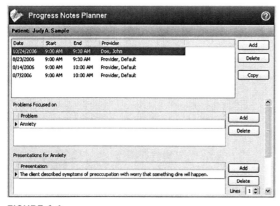

FIGURE 6.4

Progress Notes libraries include: Addiction, Adolescent, Adult, Child, Couples, Family Therapy, and Severe and Persistent Mental Illness.

New Progress Notes add-on libraries are frequently becoming available. You can visit www.therascribe.com or contact Wiley toll-free at 1-866-888-5158 for information on the latest Progress Notes add-on libraries.

Creating a Progress Note

Using the Progress Notes Planner Libraries

To quickly create a progress note using the Progress Notes Planner libraries:

1. Click **Add,** to the right of the **Problems Focused On** data grid. A library selection window will appear, listing all of the primary or secondary problems selected for the patient in the Treatment Plan section.

2. Click on one or more check boxes next to the problem or problems that have been the focus of your current therapy session with the patient. Click OK.

3. Click **Add** next to the **Presentations** data grid. The library selection window will show a drop-down list, briefly describing the **Definitions** that you previously selected for the target problem.

4. Choose a definition (symptom) that was evident in the session.

To select Intervention description statements:

1. Click **Add** button next to the **Interventions** data grid. At the top of the library window, you will see one of the anticipated Interventions selected for the target problem in the patient's treatment plan.

> **TIP**
> Progress toward objectives may be updated on the **Objectives Rating** screen regardless of which progress note method you choose to use.

> **TIP**
> The default presentations displayed are those most likely to present themselves in your patient, based on the behavioral **Definitions** you selected in the Treatment Plan section. You can choose from a broader array of possible presentations for the problem by clicking the **Show All Symptoms/ Definitions** box.

2. Use the dropdown list to **Select an Intervention.**
3. Then click the check boxes to select the notes that reflect the intervention used with the patient.
4. If you desire to review all of the intervention statements associated with the targeted problem, click the **Show All Interventions for this Problem** check box at the bottom of the **Select an Intervention** window.
5. Only the Primary Provider may see all notes; any Team Member may see the notes that he or she created.

Copying Progress Notes/Group Notes

Thera*Scribe*® allows you to create a progress note for one patient, then copy the progress note and session details to other patient records. Doing so might be particularly useful for updating the records of patients participating in psychoeducational/didactic sessions or other therapy groups; this easy and helpful tool can be a valuable timesaver.

1. Choose any group member, and follow the steps for entering Session Detail information.
2. Use the **Progress Notes Planner** screen or **Psychotherapy Notes** screen to create session notes.
3. Press the **Copy** button to the right of the **Session Details** data grid.
4. A **Select Patients to Copy Progress Data To** window will appear, allowing you to select the patient to whom the note should be copied.
5. The window will list all patients associated with the current user of Thera*Scribe*® that meet both of the following criteria:
   ▶ Have a primary or secondary problem in common with the progress note just created.

- Have been assigned to you as a Provider, Supervisor, or Team Member.

6. Click on the check boxes next to the patients' names into whose record you would like to copy the progress note and session data. Click **OK**.

7. Copying a Progress Note to another patient's record will cause an entry to be made to the Log of Patient Record Access for the given patient. That log is available for reference as a data grid on the HIPAA screen in the Personal Data group. A Comment will be placed in the log that indicates that a note has been copied by a specified provider into this record along with a date and time of copying.

Objective Rating

The **Objective Rating** screen (see Figure 6.5) allows you to rate your patient's progress toward achieving the objectives you set out on the **Objectives/Interventions** screen of the Treatment Plan. As on the other Progress group screens, the **Session** data grid will appear at the top of your screen, providing an reference point for key information.

Entering Ratings

1. By default, you will see all objectives selected for the patient. You may choose to limit the view to objectives associated with a certain problem. To do so, use the dropdown list in the middle of the screen to select a **Problem**.

2. You may assign a rating for each displayed objective by clicking in the **Rating** box behind the appropriate objective. Use the dropdown list to choose a rating: **Significant Regression, Regression, No Change, Some Progress,** or **Completed**.

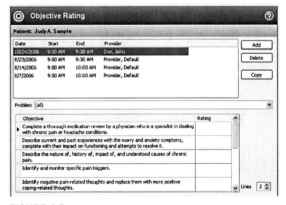

FIGURE 6.5

Being able to review quickly your patient's Objective Ratings over time will give you a helpful tool for assessing the effectiveness of the Treatment Plan. View prior progress ratings by clicking on different dates within the **Session** data grid.

3. You may use the **Objective Ratings** screen in a way that best serves your needs and work habits. Progress toward objectives may be rated sporadically, or after each session with your patient.

Psychotherapy Notes

The **Psychotherapy Notes** screen in the **Progress** group provides a narrative notes field in which you can comment on your patient's progress for each session (see Figure 6.6). You may wish to elaborate on records chosen in the Progress Notes Planner or simply make your own observations regarding the themes, symptoms, and interventions that were part of a session. Using a rich text format, you can enter an unlimited amount of information.

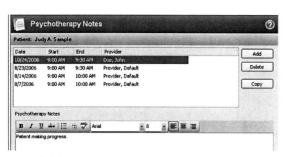

FIGURE 6.6

Entering Psychotherapy Notes:

1. Refer to the **Sessions** data grid at the top of your screen and click on the **Session** for which you would like to enter notes.
2. Click in the **Psychotherapy Notes** field and type your notes.
3. Choose a new session to enter other notes or continue work on a different screen.

Session Custom Fields

The **Session Custom Fields** screen in the **Progress** group displays specific custom fields created to record other data about sessions (see Figure 6.7).

The custom fields must be set up by the Administrator in the **Custom Fields** screen in the **Tools** group. Fields may be set up to capture text, dates,

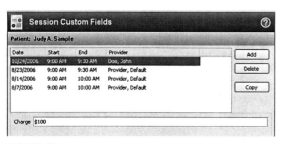

FIGURE 6.7

currency, and other types of data. The **Field Names** of the custom fields created by your system administrator are listed in the left-hand side of the screen. **Blank data** fields to capture the custom data are listed to the right of the custom field name in the **Value** column.

To enter custom data:

1. Click the **Value** field into which you want to enter data. Click **Edit,** or double-click on the blank value field.
2. A window will open, allowing entry of data through typing on the keyboard or using drop-down lists.
3. Click OK when you have finished entering your data.

Advanced users who wish to integrate the fields into appropriate sections of a Clinical Record Report may do so by customizing a report to that end (see Creating Custom Reports in the Reports section).

Amendments

The **Amendments** screen in the **Progress** group provides an important record of changes you may need to make in your patient's clinical record (see Figure 6.8). If amendments are made, you can document them here for the protection of both you and your patient.

If the locking feature has been enabled on the **HIPAA** screen in the **Tools** section, then progress notes will be locked when the user leaves the screen or switches to another patient record. Changes to notes may be made only through the **Amendments** screen.

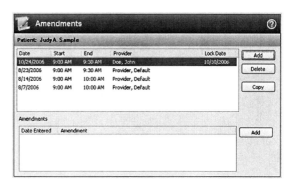

FIGURE 6.8

Making Amendments to a Patient's Record

1. Using the **Sessions** data grid at the top of your screen, select the session for which you need to add an amendment.

2. Click **Add** to the right of the **Amendments** data grid.

3. An **Amendments Entry** window will appear, allowing you to type in the amendment in a rich text format.

4. When you are ready to save your entry, click **OK.**

5. You will be prompted to confirm your entry with the following statement and question: "Once saved, amendments cannot be edited. Are you sure you want to continue?"

6. Click **Yes** to save the amendment. Click **No** to return to the **Amendments Entry** window. You can then make changes to your notes or click **Cancel.**

7. Once saved, you will have a permanent record of the amendment on file, with the **Date Entered** also noted.

CHAPTER 7

Prognosis/Discharge

| Prognosis Details | Discharge Details |

The **Prognosis/Discharge group screens** provide an overview of the treatment picture (see Figure 7.1). With the ability to review several key statistics at a glance, you can define projected levels of achievement and the time in which you hope to accomplish them with your patient. You can also plan for important components of your patient's life following the time spent in treatment with you.

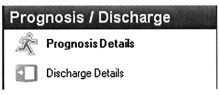

FIGURE 7.1

Prognosis Details

The **Prognosis Details** screen (see Figure 7.2) allows you to record the projected treatment outcome.

1. Objectives may be marked as critical on the **Objectives/Interventions** screen in the **Treatment Plan** group. The **Percent of Critical Objectives Required for Discharge** indicates the percent of those critical objectives that must be resolved before you can consider discharging the patient from your care. Use the dropdown list to select the percentage.

2. You can enter the **Projected Date of Treatment End,** as well as **Projected Number of Sessions Before Treatment End,** by clicking on their

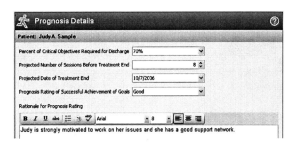

FIGURE 7.2

respective fields to type in data or by selecting from the dropdown lists.

3. Select an overall **Prognosis Rating of the Successful Achievement of Goals** from the dropdown list, which includes these ratings: **Excellent, Good, Fair, Guarded, Poor.** You may also type your own description of the prognosis into the field.

4. Looking beyond the key statistics, you can also enter a narrative rationale for your prognosis. Your insights here can be a valuable guide for yourself and your patient as you move forward with the treatment plan.

Discharge Details

The **Discharge Details** screen allows you to select criteria that must be met before your patient can be discharged from treatment (see Figure 7.3).

This screen also enables you to provide an overview of important details regarding your patient's life after discharge. You might ask: Is he competent to manage self-care and financial resources? What kind of follow-up care would best meet her needs? How will vocational plans fit in with life after treatment? The answers to these and other questions can be summarized on the **Discharge Details** screen.

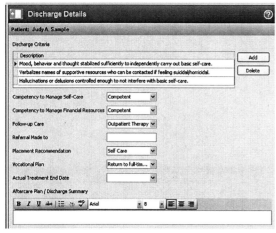

FIGURE 7.3

Creating a Plan for Aftercare and Discharge

1. Click **Add** to the right of the **Discharge Criteria** data grid. Check appropriate criteria from the **Select Discharge Criteria** window, based on your knowledge of your patient's needs and the Treatment Plan as a whole.

2. Use the dropdown lists to select relevant choices for **Competency to Manage Self-Care**

and **Competency to Manage Financial Resources** (**Competent, Competent: Needs Training, Incompetent: Can Benefit from Training, Incompetent**)

3. For **Follow-Up Care,** you can use the dropdown list to select from the following: **Community Mental Health Center, Court Services, Social Services, Substance Abuse Rehabilitation, Outpatient Rehabilitation.**

4. When you make a referral, type the name of that person or agency in the **Referral Made** field.

5. For **Placement Recommendations,** your patient may need any of the following: **Self Care, Own Family, Nursing Home, Community Residential Rehabilitation Services, Domicilary/Boarding Home,** or **Foster Care.**

6. Use the dropdown list to select a **Vocational Plan** from the following: **Return to part-time job, Return to full-time job, Seek part-time job, Seek full-time job, Sheltered Workshop.**

7. Enter the patient's **Actual Treatment End Date** using the dropdown calendar.

8. A narrative text field is available for recording a detailed **Aftercare Plan/Discharge Summary** for the patient. You can enter an unlimited amount of information in this rich text field.

CHAPTER 8

Appointment Scheduler

(for Small Practice and Enterprise Editions)

The Thera*Scribe*® 5.0 Appointment Scheduler screen (see Figure 8.1) provides an invaluable tool for you as an individual clinician and as part of a larger practice. Having an easy, efficient way to manage your schedule is key to helping you work at your full potential as a provider, and an important factor in meeting the needs of your patients.

The Thera*Scribe*® Appointment Scheduler can track your schedule, allowing you to enter patient appointments, meetings, and other commitments. As you quickly scan a day, week, or month at a glance, you can also:

▶ Gauge your workload and make appropriate adjustments
▶ Make treatment plan decisions for individual patients (e.g., frequency of sessions)
▶ Coordinate work with groups of patients and outside providers

In a practice with multiple providers, you can also track the schedules of colleagues. The Thera*Scribe*® Appointment Scheduler gives you a general overview of their schedules as well, enabling you to:

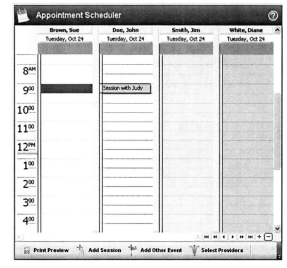

FIGURE 8.1

TIP

If you are the primary provider, supervisor, or treatment team member for a given patient, you will have access to his or her appointment schedule with other providers. Otherwise, a patient appointment will simply appear as a general note on the general calendar.

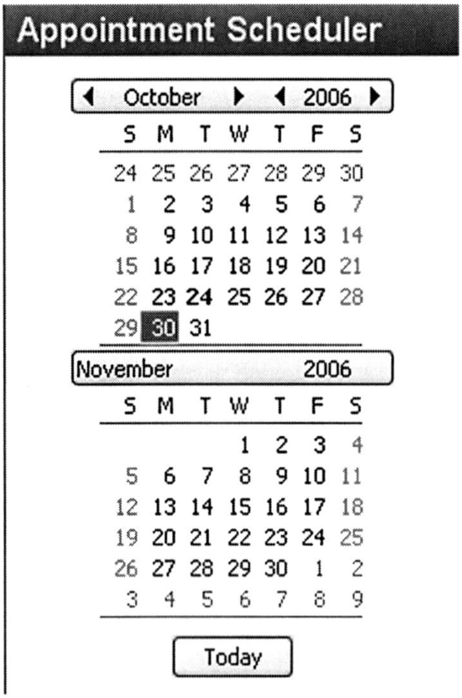

FIGURE 8.2

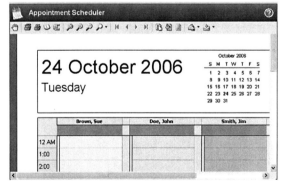

FIGURE 8.3

- Arrange for practice meetings and consultations during open time slots
- See and track sessions for patients for whom you are also responsible

The TheraScribe® Appointment Scheduler can also be used by a person responsible for scheduling appointments at your organization. This person would be designated as a Maintenance User.

Selecting a Date

You can select a specific date by using the small monthly calendar located in the upper left corner of the **Appointment Scheduler** screen (see Figure 8.2).

1. Click the date you wish to view, and a listing of that day's times and events will appear.
2. Click **Today** to be brought immediately to the current day.
3. If you would like to view a different month or year, click the left and right arrows on either side of the month and year.

Printing a Copy of Your Appointment Schedule

1. Click **Print Preview** on the Action Bar at the bottom of the **Appointment Scheduler** screen to access a view of the calendar from which you can print (see Figure 8.3).
2. Use the Print Tool Bar to make any changes you desire and then also to print a copy of the calendar for your reference.

Adding a Session

1. Click **Add Session** on the Action Bar at the bottom of the **Appointment Scheduler** screen to schedule a new session with a patient.
2. You will be brought to the **New Session** window. Use the dropdown calendars and lists to

enter **Date**, **Start** and **End Times**, **Patient Name**, **Provider,** and **Modality.** Use the check box to indicate Billable time.

3. Click **Appointment Scheduler** on the Navigation Bar to return to the **Scheduler** screen, where the new session will appear (see Figure 8.4).

Adding Other Events

1. Click **Add Other Event** on the Action Bar at the bottom of the **Appointment Scheduler** screen to schedule other appointments unrelated to patient care.
2. A **New Event** window will allow you enter data regarding personal appointments (e.g., lunch with a spouse), professional appointments (e.g., conferences and seminars), and practice-related appointments (e.g., staff development meetings) (see Figure 8.5).
3. Use the dropdown lists to select **Start Date** and **Time** and **End Date** and **Time,** or type in the dates and times.
4. Enter the **Subject** and click **All Day Event** if that applies.
5. Use the rich text box at the bottom to enter any narrative notes you wish to include about the appointment.
6. Click **OK** to add the appointment to your calendar or **Cancel** to return to the **Appointment Scheduler** screen without making the changes.

Selecting Which Providers to Include on Appointment Scheduler Screen

1. Click **Providers** on the Action Bar at the bottom of the **Appointment Scheduler** screen to select the providers whose schedules you would like to see included on this screen (see Figure 8.6). You might choose to select providers with

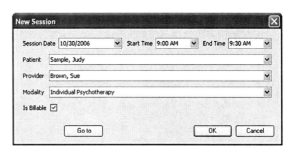

FIGURE 8.4

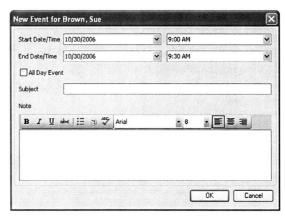

FIGURE 8.5

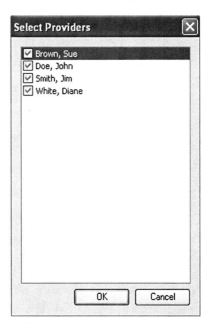

FIGURE 8.6

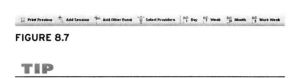

FIGURE 8.7

TIP

The more providers or days displayed at one time, the smaller the amount of space available for displaying information regarding the appointments of each. So, use this selection function to choose the display that best meets your needs at the moment.

TIP

In the **Day** view, you can select the calendar time interval by right clicking on the time display on the left.

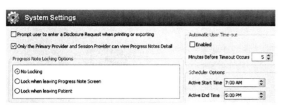

FIGURE 8.8

whom you share patients, providers with openings to whom you can refer new patients, or all providers to be included in a given staff meeting. Thera*Scribe*® flexible nature provides you with a variety of easily accessible options.

Selecting Different Views for the Appointment Scheduler Screen

1. Use the Action Bar at the bottom of the **Appointment Scheduler** screen to select a Day, Week, Month, or Work Week view (see Figure 8.7).
2. Select your choice by clicking on **Day, Week, Month,** or **Work Week.** If an option is not displayed, click the down arrow to the right of the Action Bar to see hidden options.
3. Click a new choice to change the view again.

Selecting Active Start Time and End Times

1. To select the **Active Start Time** and **Active End Time** for your day, go to the **System Settings** screen in the Tools group (see Figure 8.8).
2. Use the dropdown lists to select the desired times.

CHAPTER 9

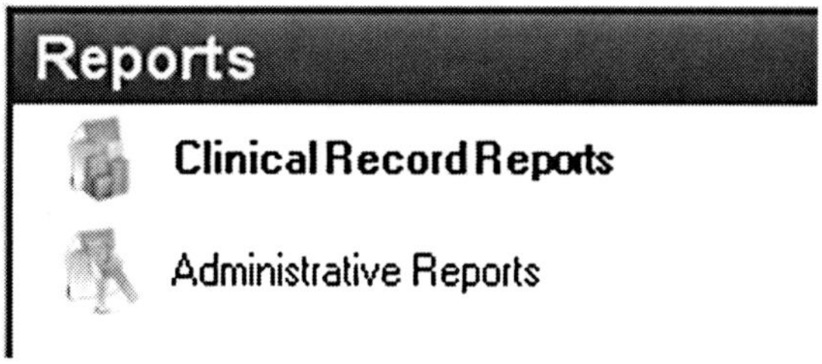

Reports

Clinical Record Reports   Administrative Reports

The Reports group screens in Thera*Scribe*® offer an array of built-in clinical records. You can choose the record that best meets your needs. The choices include:

▶ Richly formatted clinical record
▶ Lightly formatted clinical record
▶ Richly formatted concise clinical record
▶ Lightly formatted concise clinical record
▶ Session Data

You may use the **Clinical Record Report** screen to print or export clinical reports in their entirety (see Figure 9.1). You may also select which sections of the built-in clinical record reports you wish to print or export to a word processor.

The **Administrative Reports** screen includes four built-in administrative reports:

▶ Mailing labels list
▶ Patient list
▶ Provider Case Load
▶ Diagnosis History

FIGURE 9.1

Importing and Exporting Reports

You may decide to work with the Thera*Scribe*® developer or another technical specialist to create a custom report format for your patients. If you do, follow these steps to import and export reports to and from your system.

1. Go to the **Clinical Record Reports** screen or **Administrative Reports** screen, as appropriate for your custom report type.
2. To import a report, click **Add.**
3. In the **New Report** dialog box, select **Blank Report.** Click **OK.**
4. Click **Properties.** The **Report Properties** dialog box will appear.
5. Click **Import.**
6. The **Select a Thera*Scribe*® Report Template Document** dialog box will appear.
7. Type in a title for the report to be imported in the **Name** field or select it with your mouse. Click **Open** to import the report.

Exporting Reports

1. To export a report for modification by a third party, go to the **Clinical Record Reports** screen or **Administrative Reports** screen, as appropriate for your custom report type.
2. Click to highlight the report you wish to export.
3. Click **Properties.**
4. In the **Report Properties** dialog box, click **Export.**
5. In the **Thera*Scribe*® Report Document Template Export** window, type in a **File Name** for the report.

6. Choose the location to which you plan to export the report.
7. Click **Save.**

Clinical Record Reports

Choosing a Clinical Record Report Format

On the **Clinical Record Reports** screen, you can select the type of built-in clinical record report you wish to generate.

1. Select a report from the **Report** data grid by clicking on it.
   - ▶ The **Richly Formatted Clinical Record** contains an attractively designed report listing all of the fields in Thera*Scribe*®.
   - ▶ The **Richly Formatted Concise Clinical Record** features the most commonly used fields in Thera*Scribe*®.
   - ▶ The **Lightly Formatted** versions of each report are ideal for launching as RTF (rich text format) files for editing within any word processor.
   - ▶ The **Session Data** report allows for the printing of the patient's Name, Date of Report, and several pieces of objective information regarding the treatment session: Session Number, Date of Session, Start and End Time, Duration of the Session, CPT code linked to the session, treatment Modality used for the session, Provider, and overall Progress Rating entered for the session. The Session Date Filter is available for this report, allowing you to select a date or a range of dates that the report will cover.

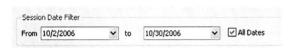

FIGURE 9.2

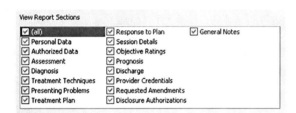

FIGURE 9.3

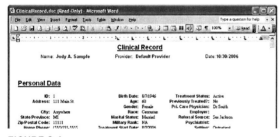

FIGURE 9.4

2. An arrow will appear in front of the report you choose to generate.

Using the Sessions Date Filter

In the **Sessions Date Filter** fields, use the dropdown calendars to select the appropriate dates for the information you plan to view (see Figure 9.2).

Viewing Selected Report Sections

You can customize your report by using the checklist at the bottom of the screen. Choices include: **Personal Data, Authorized Data, Assessment, Diagnosis, Treatment Techniques, Presenting Problems, Treatment Plan, Response to Plan, Progress Notes, Objective Ratings, Prognosis, Discharge, Provider Credentials,** and **General Notes** (see Figure 9.3).

1. By default, the (all) box and all report sections will be checked.
2. If you want to specify only certain report sections, click an item that is already selected to deselect it.

Previewing and Printing Reports

The **Preview** function allows you to see all the data you have collected and stored on various Thera*Scribe*® screens in a report form. The clinical report template you have chosen will determine the amount of data and the form in which it is presented. The clinical report will be generated for the patient name indicated near the top of your screen (see Figure 9.4).

Note: In the Trial Edition, the preview of the report is read-only and cannot be edited or printed.

1. Click **Preview** to preview the report as a document in your word processor. You can make changes and edit the report as you desire.

2. Print the report if desired.
3. Close your word processor to return to the **Clinical Record** screen.

Note: Changes that you make to clinical record reports in your word-processor version will not be stored in Thera*Scribe*®. To permanently alter report formats and contents, use the custom reports function described later in this section.

Creating Custom Reports (Small Practice and Enterprise Editions)

Users with Administrator-level security may create customized clinical or administrative report templates by adapting the built-in reports using their word processing program. If you are a novice computer user, we urge you to leave the report customization function aside until you gain complete familiarity with Thera*Scribe*®. You may then want to try your hand at a variety of customizations suggested in this section.

Note: Creating custom reports can be time-consuming and challenging for less technical users. Report customization services are available from the Thera*Scribe*® developer, PEC Technologies, LLC. Contact PEC to inquire about customization services, at their website: www.pectechnologies.com/TheraScribe or via phone email: therascribe@pectechnologies.com. Costs for report customization vary depending upon the extent of the alterations needed. You can also consult the Thera*Scribe*® website at www.therascribe.com.

You may decide that you want to add your personal touch or improve a report template to better meet the needs of your patients and practice. To customize one of the Thera*Scribe*® versions of the Clinical Record Report, you must first make a copy of the report you wish to change (see Figure 9.5).

TIP

This report and any changes you make to this document can be saved in your word processor by using the save function. However, these changes will not be made on the related Thera*Scribe*® screens.

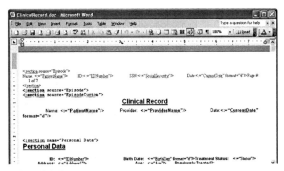

FIGURE 9.5

To make a copy:

1. Click **Add** on the **Clinical Records Reports** screen.
2. Select **Copy Existing Report** and use the drop-down list to select the report you wish to change.
3. Click **OK.**

To customize a report:

1. Select a copied report.
2. Click **Properties.**
3. Click **Edit.** The report will be opened in your word processor, where you can then make changes.
4. Click **Save** to save changes.

Importing Report Templates from a Word Processor

Sometimes you may want to import a new report template from another source (e.g. something you have purchased from a professional developer or a new layout you received at a conference) (see Figure 9.6). You can easily bring this new template into Thera*Scribe*® by using the **Clinical Reports** screen.

1. Click **Add** on the **Clinical Record Reports** screen.
2. Select **Blank Report,** as you will want to create a spot on the **Reports** data grid in which to import your new record.
3. Click **Properties.**
4. A **Report Properties** dialog box will appear. Click **Import.**
5. In the Thera*Scribe*® **Report Template Document Import** window that appears, select the report from your word processor.

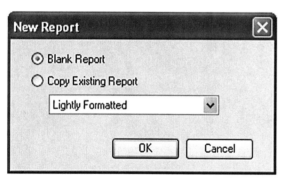

FIGURE 9.6

6. You will be asked to confirm: "Are you sure you want to overwrite the template of the selected report?" Click **Yes** to import the new report. Click **No** to return to the **Report Properties** dialog box.

Exporting Report Templates to a Word Processor

1. Select a report and click **Properties** on the **Clinical Record Reports** screen.
2. A **Report Properties** window will appear, in which you can click **Export** (see Figure 9.7).
3. In the Thera*Scribe*® **Report Template Document Export** window that appears, save the report to your word processor by giving the file a name and choosing a location in which to save it.
4. To return to Thera*Scribe*® close your word processor.

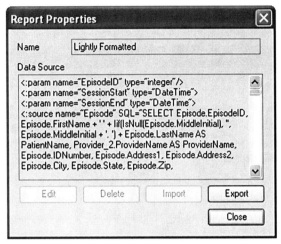

FIGURE 9.7

Administrative Reports

The **Administrative Reports** screen in the **Reports** group of Thera*Scribe*® contains four types of built-in administrative reports (see Figure 9.8):

▶ **Patient List** gives the names and treatment start dates of patients. Lists can be generated showing all patients in the database, or those meeting specific criteria (e.g., female patients, active patients, patients tied to a specific provider).

▶ **Address Labels** generates a list of addresses suitable for printing directly onto laser-printer labels (see Figure 9.9).

▶ The **Provider Case Load** report shows the current case load by provider. For each provider it shows the number of **Active Cases, Opened Cases,** and

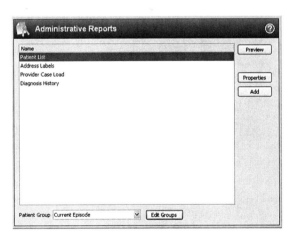

FIGURE 9.8

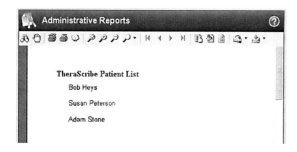

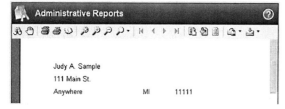

FIGURE 9.9

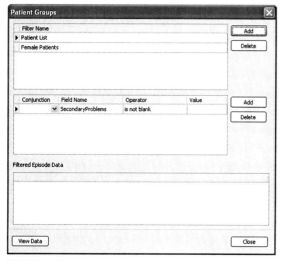

FIGURE 9.10

Closed Cases. The Active Cases are calculated by counting episodes where the specified date range overlaps the treatment start date or the treatment end date. Opened Cases are calculated by counting episodes where the treatment start date falls within the specified date range. Closed Cases are calculated by counting episodes where the treatment end date falls within the specified date range.

▶ **Diagnosis History** provides a summary of the selected patient's diagnosis history, including **Treatment Start Date, Axis, Legal Code,** and **Description.**

Generating Patient Lists and Address Labels

1. Click to highlight the type of administrative report you wish to generate.

2. Both the **Mailing Labels List** and the **Patient List** default to printing all patient records in Thera*Scribe*®.

3. To narrow the selection of patients to include on the address list or patient list, use the **Patient Group** dropdown list, where you can select certain patient groups.

4. Create new patient groups by clicking **Edit Groups.** The **Patient Group** window will appear (see Figure 9.10).

5. Use the fields in this window to assign a new Group name in the first data grid and search criteria in the center data grid. (Consult the Analyze/Compare Groups of Patients section in the Outcomes section for a detailed explanation of how to create groups of patients.)

6. Click **View Data** to generate a list of patients meeting the selected criteria.

7. Click **Close** to return to the **Administrative Reports** screen.

8. Click **Preview** to preview the report.
9. Use the **Report** Tool Bar at the top of the screen to access a variety of tools including: print, page setup, background, multiple pages, zoom, export, and send email.
10. Click on the Navigation Bar to return to the main **Administrative Reports** screen.

Generating Provider Case Load Reports

1. Click to highlight **Provider Case Load.**
2. Click **Preview** and use the dropdown calendars to enter the **Activity Start Date** and **Activity End Date** in the **Report Parameter** window (see Figure 9.11).
3. The **Provider Case Load** will display **Active Cases, Open Cases,** and **Closed Cases** (see Figure 9.12).
4. Use the Report Tool Bar at the top of the screen to access a variety of tools including: print, page setup, background, multiple pages, zoom, export, and send email.
5. Click on the Navigation Bar to return to the main **Administrative Reports** screen.

Generating a Diagnosis History Report

1. Click to highlight **Diagnosis History** (see Figure 9.13).
2. Click **Preview** to view the report, which will include **Patient Name, Treatment Start Date, Axis, Legal Code, Description, Date Added,** and **Date Deleted.**
3. Use the Report Tool Bar at the top of the screen to access a variety of tools including: print, page setup, background, multiple pages, zoom, export, and send email.
4. Click on the Navigation Bar to return to the main **Administrative Reports** screen.

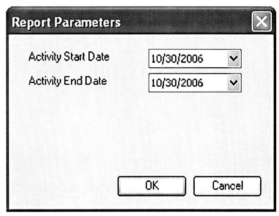

FIGURE 9.11

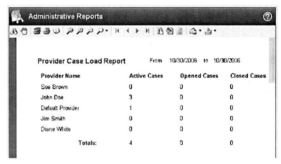

FIGURE 9.12

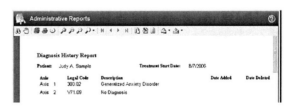

FIGURE 9.13

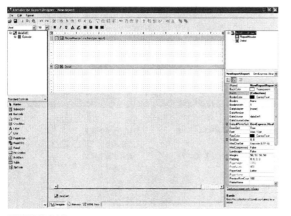

FIGURE 9.14

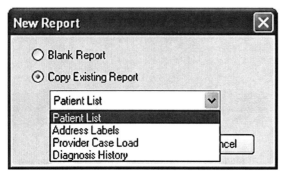

FIGURE 9.15

Advanced TIP

Administrative Reports with the option set to Custom SQL can be configured to prompt for parameter values by using parameter values in the SQL statement. Parameters should start with the @ character and contain only letters and numbers. This is an example of an SQL statement with a parameter:

SELECT*FROM Episode WHERE TreatementStartDate < @FilterDate

If a parameter names "CurrentEpisodeID" is used, then it will not be prompted for and the EpisodeID of the current episode will be used.

Creating a Custom Administrative Report

Creating customized administrative reports is somewhat less complicated than crafting custom clinical records:

1. On the **Administrative Reports** screen, click **Add**. A **New Report** dialog box will appear (see Figure 9.14).
2. Type in a **Name** for the new report.
3. If you choose to start with a blank report, check the box adjacent to "**Blank Report,**" and press **OK** to return to the administrative tab.
4. Select the report you just named, and press the **Edit** button to create the report.
5. You may copy and edit previously created custom reports by clicking the **Copy Custom Report** option and selecting a report to alter by using the dropdown menu (see Figure 9.15). To return to the **Administrative Reports** tab, press **OK**. To alter the report (e.g., change font, add or delete fields), select the newly named report and press **Edit**.

CHAPTER 10
Outcomes

| Selection Criteria | Results |

The **Outcomes group screens** (see Figure 10.1) allow you to access the Thera*Scribe*® database in order to analyze outcomes for a given patient. You may want to compare your patient to others while developing a treatment plan. You may also choose to assess your patient's progress in comparison to others as you hone your approaches or look ahead to future decisions.

The **Outcomes** group also enables you to look at groups of patients. As you proceed with treatment, you can analyze functional improvement or deterioration for a patient or group of patients meeting certain criteria that you have specified (e.g., active patients with depression treated by Dr. John Doe versus active patients with depression treated by Ms. Mary Smith).

A variety of measures are available for use in your analysis. These include: Progress Ratings, Global Assessment of Functioning (GAF) scores, Test Results, and Risk Assessment Results.

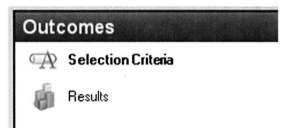

FIGURE 10.1

Selection Criteria

Selecting Specific Patients for Analysis/Comparison

1. Click **Add Episodes** to make selections for analysis.

2. The **Select Episodes for Outcomes** window will appear, allowing you to select a patient or multiple patients using the check boxes (see Figure 10.2).

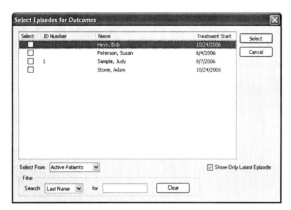

FIGURE 10.2

> **TIP**
>
> To save the given selection of patients for future reference, click **Save Criteria**. A dialog box will prompt you to **Enter the Criteria Name**.

> **TIP**
>
> If you have already set up Outcome Criteria in your previous work (descriptions of a certain selection of individuals and/or groups), you may click **Open Criteria** to view a list of these. Clicking the desired entry will then allow you to move quickly to your analysis.

3. To see more than the most recent episode for each client, click the check box by **Show Only Latest Episode**.

4. To select from **All Clients, Providers,** or **Clinical Pathways,** use the dropdown list.

5. If you choose "**Provider,**" select the name of the provider from the dropdown that appears.

6. To Search for a specific person, use the dropdown list to choose the **Field** (Last Name, First Name, ID Number) and then click to enter a value in the text box.

7. When you are satisfied with your selections, click **Select**. To exit the window without making selections, click **Cancel**.

Selecting Specific Groups for Analysis/Comparison

1. Sometimes you will want to include specific groups in your analysis, either in comparison to one another or in conjunction with your analysis of an individual.

2. Click **Add Groups** to make your selections.

3. Use the check boxes in the **Select Patient Groups** window to designate the applicable groups (see Figure 10.3).

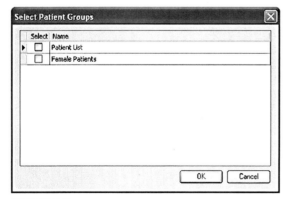

FIGURE 10.3

4. Click **OK** to return to the **Selection Criteria** screen with your selections. Click **Cancel** to exit the window without making changes.

Analyzing and Comparing Data

You can analyze a variety of data types:

- Progress ratings
- Days in treatment
- Global assessment of functioning ratings (GAF for Current, Prior, and Current vs. Prior)
- Risk assessment ratings
- Test results (for one patient at multiple points in time)
- Test results across multiple patients

  1. Use the dropdown list for **Type of Data** and click to select the type you desire (see Figure 10.4).
  2. Depending upon the Type of Data you choose to analyze, you may be prompted to select a **Statistic Calculated** (e.g., median or mean) or **Points of Comparison** (e.g., pre, post, and follow-up; multiple points in treatment) from dropdown menus.
  3. If you choose test results, use the dropdown menus to select **Instrument Group** and **Subscale,** as needed.
  4. Click **Create Results** to retrieve the data you selected for the patients chosen.

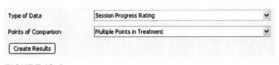

FIGURE 10.4

Adding New Groups

1. If you wish to create a new group, defined with specific criteria by which you can conduct your analysis, click **Edit Groups.**
2. The **Patients Group** window will allow you to define your new group.

TIP

If you want to focus your search, use the **AND**. If you want to broaden the field for which your criteria will apply, use the conjunction **OR**.

TIP

If you want to print out a list of the patients who meet the sort criteria you have defined, go to the **Reports/Administrative Reports** screen and select **Patient List** from the **Report Layout** box. Select the desired **Patient Group** from the dropdown list and click **Preview** to view the report. Click the printer icon at the top left of the screen to print the list.

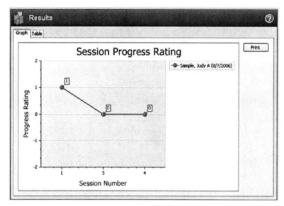

FIGURE 10.5

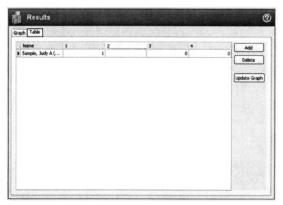

FIGURE 10.6

3. Click **Add** to the right of the **Filter Name** grid to provide a new line on which to type in the group name.

4. Once the name is entered, click **Add** to the right of the center data grid and continue by specifying several key elements:

  ▶ Conjunction ("**AND**" is the default, meaning patients who meet the criteria you are about to define as well as those in the previous row; "**OR**" can be chosen, meaning patients who meet this set of criteria or the one above, but not necessarily both)

  ▶ Field Names (e.g., Approaches, Family History, Gender, Prognosis Rating, and many more)

  ▶ Operators (e.g., equal to, less than)

  ▶ Values (e.g., specific results to search for on the selected row, such as "female" if Gender was selected)

When you have finished selecting search criteria:

1. Click **View Data** button at the bottom of the window. Patients meeting the selected criteria will be displayed in the filtered **Episode Data** grid. Each line will supply a comprehensive overview of data about a given patient.

2. Click **Create Results** to move to the **Results** screen and view the analysis of your data.

Results

The **Results** screen (see Figures 10.5 and 10.6) in the **Outcomes** group allows you to view and print graphic results for the patients and groups you select on the **Selection Criteria** screen. Thera*Scribe*® provides two helpful ways to see the results, by **Graph** and **Table**.

After choosing the selection criteria, you will automatically see a graph on the Results screen. The data will be represented by either a line graph or a bar graph, depending on the type of data.

1. Click the **Table** tab near the top of the screen to see a tabular representation of the same data. Use the tabs to move between **Table** and **Graph** screens.
2. If you would like to print the table or graph, click **Print.**

> **TIP**
>
> If you frequently search for outcomes based on the same type of data (e.g., GAF scores), you may save your criteria by clicking **Save Criteria** on the **Selection Criteria** screen. In the **Save Outcome Criteria** window, give the criteria a name, and indicate where it should be saved. Click **Save.** To retrieve and rerun those criteria, click the **Open Criteria** button, select the criteria file name, and click **Open.**

CHAPTER 11

Tools

Providers	Shortcut Bar	Database
Teams/Groups	Libraries	System Settings
Custom Fields	Treatment Planners	Preferences
Default Settings	Progress Note Planners	

The Tools group screens provide a comprehensive, efficient way for you to manage customizations throughout Thera*Scribe*®, thereby allowing you to maximize the benefits of the program for your practice.

Some of the many functions available in the **Tools** group include:

▶ Making changes to the listing of Providers and key data about each

▶ Editing Treatment Teams and Groups

▶ Creating Custom Fields throughout Thera*Scribe*® to tailor the screens for your unique needs

▶ Setting Defaults for certain screens where you often enter the same data

▶ Customizing your Shortcut Bar

▶ Planning custom Treatment Plans for quick and easy future use

▶ Preparing custom Progress Notes for recurring problems in your patients

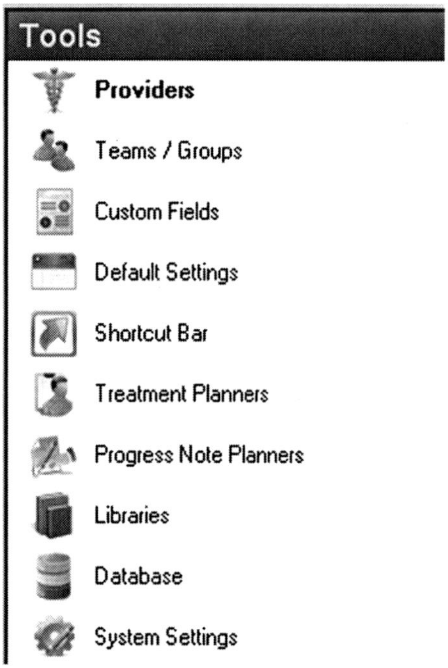

106 APPLICATION SCREENS

FIGURE 11.1

FIGURE 11.2

- Editing Dropdown Lists and Other Libraries not related to Practice Planner modules
- Managing the import and export of content from your Database
- Prescribing System Settings related to privacy issues.
- Setting preferences related to the Home Page and Appointment Scheduler.

The **Tools** group screens (see Figure 11.1) are intended to be used by the Thera*Scribe*® Administrator. It is accessible only to users who are assigned Administrator or Advanced level security on the **Providers** screen in this group. The users assigned the Maintenance level of security may be allowed access to the **Database** screen in this section only if this access is enabled on the **System Settings** screen.

Providers

The **Providers** screen in the **Tools** group allows you to enter the names of providers who will be adding data to Thera*Scribe*® for their patients (see Figure 11.2).

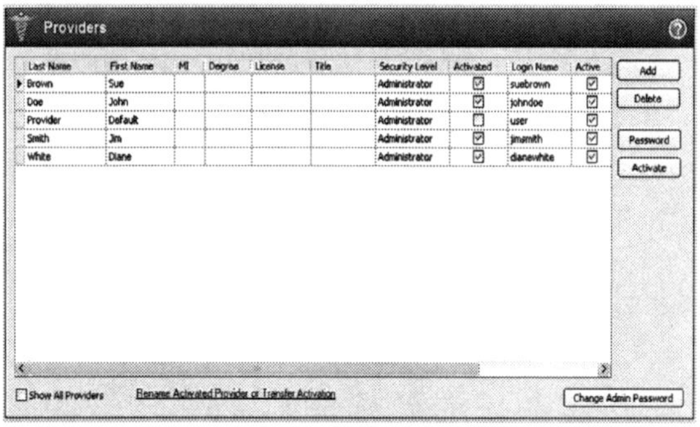

Only an Administrator may add new providers to the program, or edit the data pertaining to existing providers.

Adding New Providers

1. To add a new provider click **Add**. This will create a new line in the data grid.
2. Click on each field in the data grid to type in the new provider's Last Name, First Name, Middle Initial, Degree, License number, and the State that issued the license, and Title (or profession).

Setting User Security Levels

Click in the **Security Level** field in the **Provider** data grid to select one of four security levels (see Figure 11.3):

▶ The **Administrator** level allows the user to have complete control over all functions of Thera*Scribe*®.

FUNCTIONS	ADMINISTRATOR	ADVANCED	BASIC	MAINTENANCE
Edit provider data	All	Self	Self	Self
Change provider passwords	All	Self	Self	Self
Can select any patient	✔			✔
See data for all patients	✔			
See data for Supervisee patients + patients for whom provider is Team Member	✔	✔	✔	
View names of patients in sessions on the Appointment Scheduler	All	Only for patients the user can select	Only for patients the user can select	All
View the Access Log history	All	Only if the primary provider	Only if the primary provider	
Create or Edit Clinical Pathways	✔			
Delete Episodes	✔			
Edit libraries	✔	✔		
Create or Edit teams / groups	✔			
Create custom fields	✔			
Enter default settings	✔			
Set Authorized Session warnings	✔			
Import Planner libraries	✔			
Export or Import clinical records	✔			
Create or Edit custom reports	✔			
Create or Edit patient groups	✔			
Activate a provider	✔			

FIGURE 11.3

- The **Advanced** user setting should be used for providers to whom you wish to give the ability to permanently alter libraries.
- The **Basic** user is prevented from altering Thera*Scribe*® libraries.
- The **Maintenance** level user is able to access only the **Demographics, Provider,** and **Insurance** screens in the **Personal Data** group. In addition, this user may be given access to the **General Notes, Attachments,** and **Custom Fields** screens in the **Personal Data** group and the **Database** screen in the **Tools** group. This access is enabled on the **HIPAA** screen in the **Tools** group.

See Figure 11.3 for a list of the functions users with each of the security levels can access.

Setting Login Names and Provider Status

In the **Provider** data grid, click in the **Login Name** field and type in a 4- to 15-character name that the user will use to sign in to the program.

1. Indicate whether the provider is **Active** or **Inactive.** The check box will default to the active position for newly added providers.
2. If a provider leaves the practice, the status should be rendered inactive by unchecking the box.

Being marked **Inactive** will remove the provider's name from the **Providers** data grid as well as the **Provider** dropdown lists throughout the program. Check **Show All Providers** to include inactive providers in the **Providers** data grid and dropdown lists.

Creating and Changing Passwords

1. In the **Provider** data grid, click the name of the provider whose password is to be added or changed (see Figure 11.4).

TIP

If a provider leaves the practice, his/her patients can be reassigned to a new provider. After the name and credentials of a new provider are entered by the Administrator through the **Providers** screen, the patient may be reassigned to a different provider through the patient's **Personal Data/Provider** screen. Click the dropdown list for **Primary Provider** and select the name of the new provider. After all of the exiting provider's active patients have been reassigned in this way, mark the exiting provider as **Inactive** in the **Tools/Edit Provider** screen.

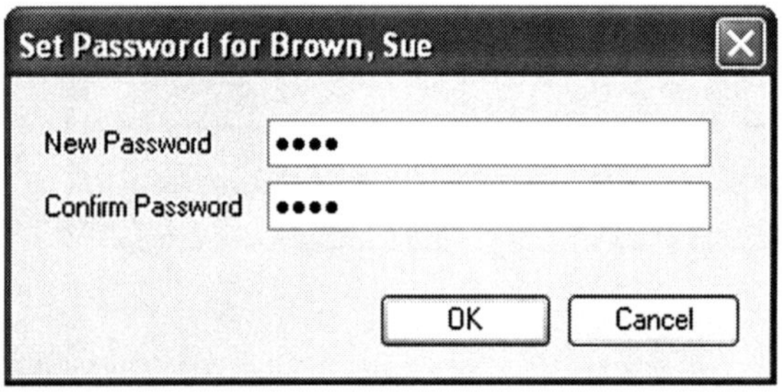

FIGURE 11.4

2. Click **Password** to the right of the data grid. A **Change Provider Password** window will appear.

   3. Type in the new password and a confirmation of it.

Changing the Administrator Password

   1. The system administrator may change his/her password by clicking **Change Admin Password** at the bottom right corner of the screen. A **Change Admin Password** window will appear.

   2. Type in the new password and a confirmation of it.

Activating a New Provider in Thera*Scribe*®

   1. Click **Activate** to the right of the **Provider** data grid to open the Thera*Scribe*® Activation Wizard (see Figure 11.5).

   2. You will be prompted with the question: "Have you purchased a license for Thera*Scribe*®?" Click **Yes** or **No** and then click **Next**.

   3. If you click **Yes,** the Activation Wizard will prompt you to enter the registration code.

   4. If you click **No,** the Activation Wizard will provide you with the phone number and website information for purchasing a Thera*Scribe*® license. Click **OK** to return to the **Provider** screen.

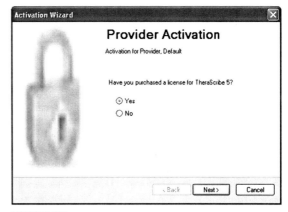

FIGURE 11.5

Changing Provider Activation

If you wish to change a provider's name or transfer activation to another provider:

   1. Click the link at the bottom of the **Provider** screen: **Rename Activated Provider** or **Transfer Activation.**

   2. The **Change Provider Activation Wizard** will be opened. Click to select one of two choices:

110 APPLICATION SCREENS

Rename Activated Provider or Transfer Activation

TIP

You can assign your patients to specific **Treatment Teams** or **Therapy Groups** on the **Provider** screen in the **Personal Data** group. Similarly, once a treatment team or therapy group has been set up (e.g., given a name and had providers assigned to it) in the **Tools** section, that team or group may be chosen for a specific patient on the **Provider** screen.

When working in the **Progress** group, you may want to copy **Progress Notes, Objective Ratings, Psychotherapy Notes,** or **Amendments** to other patient records. If you have assigned a patient to a treatment team or therapy group, his or her name will be among those displayed in the **Select Patients** window when you click **Copy.** This provides a quick and easy way to apply records of group work to several patients at once.

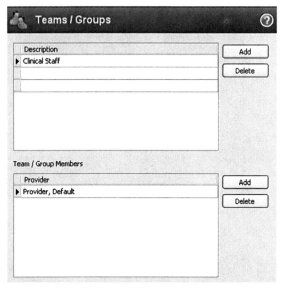

FIGURE 11.6

Rename an Existing Provider or **Transfer Activation to Another Provider.**

3. If you choose **Rename an Existing Provider,** click **Next,** select a provider from the dropdown list, and enter the new information. Click **Next** and you will be prompted to enter the **Provider Maintenance Code** to complete the process.

4. If you choose **Transfer Activation,** click **Next,** and use the dropdown lists to make the changes. Click **Next** and you will be prompted to enter the **Provider Maintenance Code** to complete the process.

Teams/Groups

The **Teams/Groups** screen in the **Tools** group allows the Administrator to do two important tasks:

▶ Set Therapy Group names (e.g., Depression)
▶ Create Treatment Teams (multiple providers with access to see and update a patient record)

Adding Group Names and Provider Teams/Groups

If you are designating a new group (see Figure 11.6):

1. Click **Add** to the right of the **Description** data grid.
2. Enter the name of the new group.
3. Click **Add** to the right of the **Team/Group Members** data grid.
4. In the **Select Team Members** window, use the check boxes to select all the providers who will be servicing the Group named above. These may be leaders of the therapy group or members of the treatment team.

5. Click **OK** or **Cancel** to return to the **Teams/Groups** screen.

Custom Fields

The **Custom Fields** screen in the **Tools** group allows for the creation of an unlimited number of customized fields in which you can collect data that may be unique to the needs of your practice (see Figure 11.7 and 11.8).

The fields that are created within this screen are available for input on the Custom Fields screen in the Personal Data group.

Creating a Custom Field

1. Select the **Field Class** (**Episode** or **Session**) using the dropdown list.
2. To create a custom field, click **Add** to the right of the data grid. A blank row will appear in the data grid.
3. Click in the **Name** column and type in the label for the custom field.
4. Click in the **Type** column and select the type of data to be entered in the field. The following table provides you with more information about the types of data.
5. Click in the **Category** column and select a desired category, then **Description.** This allows you to organize your custom fields (i.e. billing, personal info).
6. Click **Category** to the right of the grid to add a new category.

Default Settings

The **Default Settings** screen (see Figure 11.9) in the **Tools** group allows the Administrator to enter

TIP

An Administrator may add names of providers to a treatment team or therapy group leadership at any time by selecting them in the **Team/Group Members** data grid. Click **Add** to the right of the **Providers** data grid to add names. Click **Delete** to remove names.

TYPE OF DATA	FUNCTION PROVIDED
Choice	Creates dropdown lists in which you can include your choice of selections.
Currency	Displays numbers in dollars/cents
Date	Creates a dropdown calendar
Date/Time	Indicates both date and time
Number	Requires the user to enter a whole number
Text	Creates narrative text field of unlimited length
Time	Displays hours/ minutes
Yes/No	Prompts the user to select "yes" / "no"

FIGURE 11.7

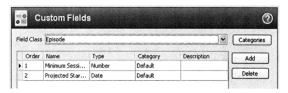

FIGURE 11.8

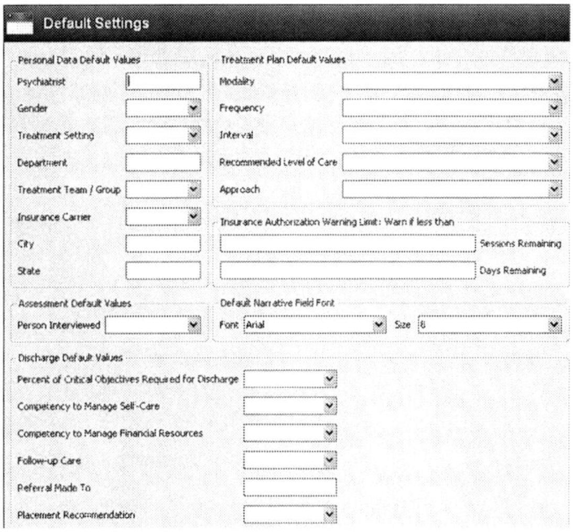

FIGURE 11.9

TIP

As a provider, you may override defaults at any time by making a new selection from a dropdown list or typing in your own text.

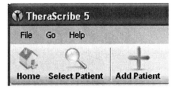

FIGURE 11.10

default values for a variety of fields within Thera*Scribe*®. If you find yourself entering data that is often repeated from one new patient to another, you can save work and time by using these default values, instead of retyping the data each time.

Some of the areas in which you can take advantage of default settings include:

▶ Personal Data (e.g., Gender, Treatment Setting, State of residence)

▶ Treatment Plan (e.g., Modality, Frequency, Approach)

▶ Insurance Authorization Warning Limit (Sessions or Days Remaining)

▶ Default Narrative Field Font (Font and Size)

▶ Discharge (e.g., Follow-Up Care, Placement Recommendation, Vocational Plan)

When you are ready to enter default values:

1. Click in the field of your choice and either choose from a dropdown list, if available, or type in your own text.

2. Selections you make on the **Default Settings** screen will then automatically appear when a clinical record is created for a new patient.

Shortcut Bar

The **Shortcut Bar** window (see Figure 11.10) allows you to customize your Shortcut Bar, located near the top of your Thera*Scribe*® screen. If you choose this **Tools** group window, you may choose to add any of nearly fifty shortcut buttons to your Shortcut Bar. As you select the buttons that link you to your most commonly used screens and functions, you will make your work processes easier and more efficient.

To make changes to your Shortcut Bar:

1. Make a selection from the list of **Available Shortcuts** by clicking on it.
2. Click **Add** to the right of this list to add it to your Shortcut Bar. Click **Remove** to remove it from your Shortcut Bar.
3. Use the **Move Up** or **Move Down** buttons to arrange the list of **Selected Shortcuts** in an order that works best for you.
4. Click **Apply** to make the changes or simply exit the screen. Click **Cancel** to cancel any changes made.

Libraries

The **Libraries** screen (see Figure 11.11) in the **Tools** group allows users with Administrator-level or Advanced-level security to permanently change the contents of the libraries not related to the add-on Practice Planner library modules. This can be done by editing, adding, or deleting options from the libraries. Some of these libraries are used in dropdown lists.

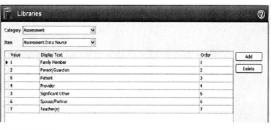

FIGURE 11.11

Editing Libraries

Library categories that may be permanently edited by Administrators from this screen include:

▶ Recovery Dimensions (Severity, Level of Care, Stage of Change)

▶ Assessment (Data Source, Assessments, Person Interviewed, Risk Level, Strengths, Treatment Phase, Weaknesses)

- ▶ Demographics (Gender, Marital Status, Race, Setting)
- ▶ Discharge (Competencies, Discharge Care, Follow-up Care, Percent Objectives, Placement Recommendation, Prognosis Rating)
- ▶ HIPAA Items (Amendment Reason for Denial, Data Section, Disclosure Purpose, Information Disclosed)
- ▶ Mental Status (Affect, Appearance, Attitude, General Knowledge, Immediate Memory, Insight, Intelligence)
- ▶ Other (Insurance, Medication Type, Medications, Modalities, Progress Rating)
- ▶ Treatment Plan (Approaches, Axis V, Complete Axis I and II Libraries, ICD-9 Diagnoses, Modality Interval, Recommended Level of Care)

1. Use the down arrow to select from **Library** you wish to edit.
2. Click **Add** button to add a new row to the library.
3. To Delete content from the library, click on the row you wish to delete, and click **Delete**.

Note: Changes made to libraries are permanent. For that reason, use caution in deleting content from the built-in libraries or add-on Practice Planner libraries.

Treatment Planners

The **Treatment Planners** screen (see Figure 11.12) in the **Tools** group allows users with Administrator level or Advanced level security to permanently change the contents of the library items. This screen allows you to enter custom treatment planner options, delete or edit built-in options,

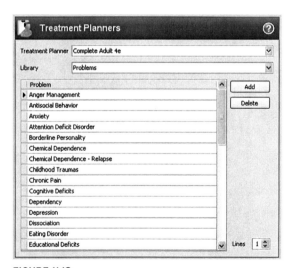

FIGURE 11.12

and add or change links between objectives and interventions.

Editing Planner Libraries

1. Use the **Treatment Planner** dropdown list to select the Treatment Planner add-on module you wish to edit.
2. Use the **Library** dropdown list to select the component you wish to change.
3. The available components include:
   - Problem
   - Definition
   - Goals
   - Objectives/Interventions
   - Axis I diagnoses
   - Axis II diagnoses
4. To add a new problem to a Treatment Planner library, choose **Problem** in the Library dropdown list.
5. To edit or add content to the libraries (e.g., Definitions, Goals, Objectives/Interventions) of an existing problem, use the **Problem** dropdown list to choose from the list of problems tied to the **Planner** you selected.
6. Use the **Lines** toggle box to increase or decrease the number of rows visible for each library item.
7. To **Edit** an existing library component, click on the row containing that item, and type in the edited content.
8. Add new content to the library component by clicking **Add** and typing the content into the blank row which appears.
9. In the **Objectives/Interventions** section, you may relate a new intervention to an existing or

new objective or edit existing links by clicking **Change** at the bottom of the screen. Check the boxes adjacent to the objective(s) you wish to tie to that intervention.

Note: Beware! If you delete a Problem, you will delete all Definitions, Goals, Objectives, Interventions, and Diagnoses associated with that problem.

Progress Note Planners

The **Progress Note Planners** screen (see Figure 11.13) in the Tools group allows users with Administrator level or Advanced level security to permanently change the contents of the Progress Note Planner library items. This screen allows you to enter custom progress note planner options and delete or edit built-in options.

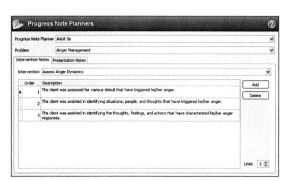

FIGURE 11.13

1. Use the **Progress Note Planner** dropdown list to select the planner you wish to change.
2. Use the **Problem** dropdown list to select a problem.
3. The **Intervention Notes** tab will display the notes typically associated with the problem; use the **Intervention** dropdown list to view notes associated with each intervention.
4. Click **Add** if you want to enter an additional custom note.
5. A new line will appear on the data grid, where you can type in your custom note.
6. Click the **Order** column heading in the data grid to reverse the given order of notes.
7. Select a note and click **Delete** to delete it from the data grid.
8. Click the **Presentation Notes** tab to view the notes typically associated with the selected problem.

9. Use the Definition dropdown list to select the **Definition** you want to change.
10. Follow steps 4–7 above to make changes to either the **Symptom Subgroup** data grid or the **Presentation Note** data grid.

Database

The **Database** screen (see Figure 11.14) in the **Tools** group provides several options for managing your Thera*Scribe*® database.

▶ The Administrator can import additional modules into Thera*Scribe*® and perform routine database maintenance.

▶ You can also use this screen to export all clinical records to an external database or statistical package, or save a single patient's clinical record to a floppy disk or other storage media.

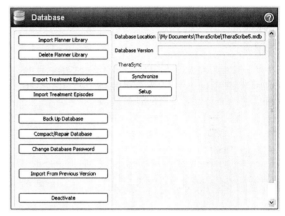

FIGURE 11.14

Importing Planner Add-On Modules

1. To import data from a new Treatment Planner, Homework Planner, or Progress Notes Planner, click **Import Planner Library** on the **Database** screen. An **Open** window will appear.
2. Browse for the file you wish to import, and click **Open.**
3. Thera*Scribe*® will copy the data from the disk into the database and make it available to the user of Thera*Scribe*®.
4. The title of the new Planner module will be displayed in the relevant dropdown lists throughout the program.

Deleting Planner Libraries

1. To delete a Planner Library, click **Delete Planner Library.**
2. In the **Delete Planner** window, use the dropdown lists to select **Planner Type** and **Planner**

title. Click **OK** to delete or cancel to return to the **Database** screen.

Exporting and Importing Clinical Records

Recognizing that many users use both desktop and laptop computers, Thera*Scribe*® provides for exchange of patient records between multiple installations of the program.

Due to data integrity requirements of most health care systems, this functionality is available only to an Administrator.

To export a patient record to your hard drive or to a writeable CD/DVD:

1. Click **Export Treatment Episode.**
2. From the **Select Episodes to Export** window, check the episode or episodes of care for a patient or group of patients that you wish to export. Click **Select.**
3. A **Save Export File** window will appear. Select the location where you want to save the episode. Type the file name (e.g., John) in the **File Name** box. Click **Save** to save the file, where it can be opened in another installation of the software using step 4.
4. Click **Import Treatment Episode** to access data saved to a hard drive or writeable CD/DVD. Locate the file in the **Look In** box. Click **Open.** This will import the file into Thera*Scribe*®, and write over earlier episodes stored in the database.

Backing Up, Repairing, and Restoring the Database

For security and data integrity reasons, you will want to make a copy of your clinical records regularly. Use the following steps to back up the Thera*Scribe*® 5.0 database:

1. To make a copy of the database, click **Back Up Database.**

TIP

The export and import patient records features operate by completely writing over the existing patient record for the specified episode of care with the most recently dated record. This functionality should be used with care, as there is no way to undo the write-over once a new episode has been imported.

2. Select the location where you want to save the backup file.
3. Type in the name of the file. Click **OK.**

If you have a backup file and want to run from that backup database:

1. Open Thera*Scribe*® 5.0.
2. Do not login to Thera*Scribe*® 5.0.
3. Click on **Open Database File.**
4. Click on **Open an Existing Database File.**
5. Find the backup database you want to run and open that file.
6. Once you are back to the login screen, you can login. Doing so will load the backup database.

To reorganize and speed access to your database, click **Compact/Repair Database.**

Changing the Database Password

The Essential® and Small Practice® Editions store data in an Microsoft Access® database that can be opened and examined using Microsoft Access®. The database comes password protected. The default password is: TS5master. The Administrator can change this password to allow access to the raw data in the database using the **Change Database Password** button. If the password is changed to a blank value, no password will be required to open it in Microsoft Access®.

Importing from a Previous Version

To import a database from Thera*Scribe*® 4.0:

1. Click **Import** from a Previous Version.
2. The Import from Thera*Scribe*® 4.0 Wizard will appear, prompting you through the steps.
3. Select either the **Solo/Small Group Version** or the **Enterprise SQL Version.**

4. Enter either the **Database File** or **Server** name.
5. Click **Next**.
6. Continue working through the Wizard.

Note: All patient and session data is imported except the following: the admin account password, TheraSync settings, Administration/HIPAA data, Administration/Default Settings data, Saved Outcome Criteria, and any Report Layouts.

Note: If a particular Planner Library has been loaded into Thera*Scribe*®, and the Planner is also in the Thera*Scribe*® 4.0 data being imported, it will be skipped. This includes any changes made to the Planner. Otherwise, the Planner with changes will be imported.

Deactivating Thera*Scribe*®

1. If you wish to deactivate the current version of Thera*Scribe*® and return to Trial Mode, click **Deactivate**.
2. You will be asked to confirm your desire to deactivate by clicking **Yes**. Click **No** to return to the **Database** screen.

Using TheraSync®

TheraSync® is designed to synchronize the Therapist Helper™ and Thera*Scribe*® software applications and allow for data exchange between the two. After some initial setup, TheraSync® operates from a single Synchronize button on the **Database** screen in Thera*Scribe*®. If you are part of a larger office you will probably want to synchronize at least once a week to ensure that any new patient and/or provider information is identical in both applications. Still larger offices may need to synchronize more often.

▶ Preparing for Initial Setup

TheraSync® synchronizes three sets of data between Therapist Helper™ and TheraScribe®: patients, providers, and sessions. Each one of these sets requires its own setup in order for TheraSync® to know how to handle the data.

▶ Setting Up TheraSync®

1. Open TheraScribe® and go to the **Database** screen in the **Tools** group. Click **Setup.**

2. In the TheraSync® setup window, use the **Application** dropdown list to select **Therapist Helper**™.

3. Click and complete the **Patient** tab data based on the following values:

   a) Automatically look for matching new records in TheraScribe® and Therapist Helper™. Check this box if you want TheraSync® to match records based on patient name. For example, if TheraSync® finds a patient named Smith, John in both Therapist Helper™ and TheraScribe®, it marks the patient as a match between the two applications. If you do not have this box checked, you must do the matching manually. We recommend that this option be left on; otherwise duplicate data may start appearing in Therapist Helper™ when synchronizing multiple times.

   b) Conflict Resolution. If TheraSync® finds mismatched data between matched records in Therapist Helper™ and TheraScribe®, you must decide how it will handle the resolution. Select one of three options:

   Use TheraScribe® Value: Therapist Helper™ is overwritten with the data from TheraScribe®.

Use Therapist Helper™ Value: TheraScribe® is overwritten with the data from Therapist Helper™.

Do Nothing: TheraScribe® and Therapist Helper™ remain as they are; neither application is overwritten with data from the other.

c) New Records. If new records have been added to either application, you can select to transfer that new data to the other application. For example, if you add a new patient to Therapist Helper™, you can select **Add** new records found in Therapist Helper™ to TheraScribe® to have that patient transferred to TheraScribe® and vice versa.

4. Click and complete the **Provider** tab data based on the following values:

a) Automatically look for matching new records in TheraScribe® and Therapist Helper™. Check this box if you want TheraSync® to match records based on provider name. For example, if TheraSync® finds a provider named Smith, Jane in both Therapist Helper™ and TheraScribe®, it marks the provider as a match between the two applications. If you do not have this box checked, you must do the matching manually.

b) Conflict Resolution: If TheraSync® finds mismatched data between matched records in Therapist Helper™ and TheraScribe®, you must decide how it will handle the resolution. Select one of three options:

Use TheraScribe® Value: Therapist Helper™ is overwritten with the data from TheraScribe®.

Use Therapist Helper™ Value: Thera-Scribe® is overwritten with the data from Therapist Helper™.

Do Nothing: TheraScribe® and Therapist Helper™ remain as they are; neither application is overwritten with data from the other.

c) New Records: If new records have been added to either application, you can select to transfer that new data to the other application. For example, if you add a new provider to Therapist Helper™, you can select **Add** new records found in Therapist Helper™ to TheraScribe® to have that provider transferred to TheraScribe®, and vice versa.

5. Click and complete the Sessions tab data based on the following:

a) Automatically look for matching new records in TheraScribe® and Therapist Helper™. This box is grayed out for Sessions. TheraSync® automatically looks for matches between sessions.

b) Conflict Resolution: follow same guidelines as for Patients and Providers.

c) New Records: follow same guidelines as for Patients and Providers.

6. Click the **Other Options** tab to enter miscellaneous setup items:

a) Debug Mode. This may be useful for troubleshooting problems.

b) Filter Sessions. This allows you to filter sessions to those added since the last synchronization. This can greatly reduce the time required to import data if there are many session to review.

7. Click **OK** to complete the TheraSync® setup process.

Running the Synchronization

Once you have TheraSync® set up to handle the data sets between Therapist Helper™ and Thera*Scribe*®, you are ready to run the synchronization. TheraSync® first examines the data, then matches like elements, either automatically or manually according to your setup, before doing the final synchronization.

To run TheraSync®:

1. Go to the **Database** screen in the **Tools** group.
2. Click **Synchronize.** The **Examining Data** dialog box appears. If you need to do any matching or unmatching, click **Modify** next to any of the three update areas to change the synchronized information. (These steps are described in more detail under the next section: To Match/Unmatch Records.)
3. Click **Do Update** to finalize the synchronization.
4. Click **Yes** to confirm the changes.
5. Click **OK** to complete the synchronization.

To Match Records

If you need to do any matching from the Synchronize Information window:

1. Click **Modify** next to any of the three update areas. For example, if you prefer to match patients manually, you can uncheck the **Automatically look for matching new records** in Thera*Scribe*® and Therapist Helper™ box under the **Patient** setup tab, run the **Synchronization** process, and then go into the **Modify** panel.

2. To **Match,** highlight a name in the **Unmatched** in Thera*Scribe*® box and the **Unmatched** in Therapist Helper™ column and click **Match.** These records move to the **Matched Items** box and are now linked in TheraSync®.

3. To **Remove Match,** highlight a line in the **Matched Items** section and click **Remove Match.** These records are split apart in TheraSync® and move to the respective **Unmatched** columns.

To Unmatch Records

1. Click on an item in the **Unmatched** lists to view more details on the item.
2. Click **Next.**
3. The **Unmatched Patients** screen appears. (The term "**Unmatched**" means that the patient does not appear in the corresponding application. For example, if Henry Fonda appears in the Unmatched Patients in Thera*Scribe*® column, it means that Henry Fonda does not appear in Therapist Helper™. That particular patient is an "**Unmatched**" state in Thera*Scribe*®.)
4. Double click on an item here to view more detail.
5. Check the corresponding boxes according to the following definitions:
   ▶ Checked: The patient will be added as a new patient in the corresponding application.
   ▶ Grayed: No action will be taken for this patient. when you run the synchronization again, this patient will appear once more.
   ▶ Unchecked: The patient will be marked as inactive in the existing application. By design, neither application deletes patients.
6. Click **Next.**

7. The **Resolve Mismatches** screen appears. This screen shows the field-level detail of any outstanding mismatches, allowing you to select the precise information to copy over to the corresponding application. For example, if a patient's phone number shows an incorrect area code in Therapist Helper™, you can select the value in Thera*Scribe*® to carry over to Therapist Helper™.

8. Check the boxes next to the values that you want to use in both systems, or click the **Select All** buttons to copy over all values for a particular application.

System Settings

The **System Settings** screen (see Figure 11.15) in the Tools group gives the Administrator access to several functions within the program that are related to meeting the requirements of the Federal HIPAA regulations effective in April 2003. Although these functions do not make the provider HIPAA-compliant in and of themselves, they do provide prompts and assistance for making compliance more easily attained. The **Systems Settings** screen also allows the Administrator to select **Active Start Time** and **End Time** for the **Appointment Scheduler.** Changes on this screen will apply to all users.

Disclosure Request Check Box

▶ If you want a disclosure authorization prompt to be displayed every time a report is going to be printed, check the **Disclosure Request** check box.

▶ Any attempt to print a report of clinical data from the **Reports** screen will prompt a dialog box to appear which contains a reminder that

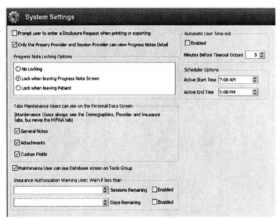

FIGURE 11.15

disclosure authorization is necessary before any information can be shared. The dialog box allows the user to indicate that he or she would like to enter disclosure authorization information and, if so, a second data entry dialog box appears.

Progress Note Detail Check Box

▶ Clicking this box allows for all the **Progress Note** (**Progress Notes Planner, Objective Rating, Psychotherapy Notes,** and **Amendments**) to be seen by only the Primary Provider assigned to the patient on the **Provider** screen in the **Personal Data** section. It allows a Team Member assigned to the patient to view only notes that he or she has entered. When this box is unchecked all Progress Notes may be viewed by any provider who is assigned to the patient.

Progress Note Locking Options Check Boxes

The **Progress Note Locking Options** check boxes allow the Administrator to select one of three options:

▶ No Locking of notes
▶ Lock when leaving the **Progress** screen
▶ Lock when leaving **Patient**

When a progress note is locked it may never be edited or deleted. The name of provider who created the note is locked along with the date of entry. This will add the **Amendment** screen to the **Progress** group. The **Amendment** screen allows the user to enter a change to the note through the entry of amendment text. This text is also locked and not able to be edited or deleted after the user leaves the screen or selects a new patient.

Maintenance User Check Boxes

In the next set of check boxes, the administrator may select what screens **Maintenance Users** are able to access in the **Personal Data** group in addition to Demographics, Provider, and Insurance. The other screen options are:

- General Notes
- Attachments
- Custom Fields

The next check box indicates whether the Maintenance User is allowed to see the Database screen in the Tools group.

Insurance Authorization Warning Limit Settings

Use the dropdown lists to select settings for sessions remaining and days remaining data. Use the check boxes to enable or disable the **Insurance Authorization Warning Limit** settings.

Automatic User Time-Out Function

- To help protect confidential PHI from being viewed by unauthorized persons, the **Automatic User Time-out** function may be enabled by checking the box provided. By entering a number in the **Minutes Before Time-out Occurs** box, you are setting the time after which the monitor screen will go blank if no activity occurs within the program.
- If the user leaves the screen unattended for the established number of minutes, the screen will go blank, protecting the patient information from being seen or the program from being operated by unauthorized people who might gain access to confidential information.

▶ The user who last logged on must enter his or her system password to unlock the blank screen and return the program to full functioning status.

Appointment Scheduler Options

You may want to change the Active Start and End Times of your practice day. Using the dropdown lists to change these times will change the start and end times for the Appointment Scheduler.

Preferences

Setting Home Page Preferences

You can set the number of Recently Selected Episodes and Upcoming Appointments that appear on your Home Screen in Thera*Scribe*® by using the **Preferences** screen in the **Tools** group (see Figure 11.16). Use the dropdown lists to make your selection or type in the number you desire.

Setting Time Interval for the Appointment Scheduler

You can also set the time interval that will appear on your Appointment Scheduler by using the dropdown list on the **Preferences** screen in the **Tools** group.

Opening the Log Folder

If an error occurs while you are using Thera*Scribe*®, an error file will be created. This file will be stored in a special directory called the **Log Folder**. To access error files:

1. Click **Open Log Folder.**
2. Select an error file.
3. You can then view the file or send the file to technical support for diagnostic work.

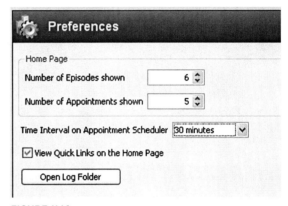

FIGURE 11.16

Technical Support

If you have Thera*Scribe*®-related questions, Technical Support Representatives may be contacted on the web at www.therascribe.com, via phone by dialing (800)762-2974 (United States only). Hours of availability are 8:00 AM to 8:00 PM Eastern time, excluding weekends and holidays. International callers may use 1-317-572-3994. If you have Therapist Helper™ questions, please call 1-781-937-0080 Monday through Friday 9:00 AM to 5:00 PM Eastern time. Depending on the issue you are encountering, you may be referred to the other product's support department.

License Agreement

SOFTWARE LICENSE AGREEMENT

Important—Read carefully before opening software package.

This is a legal agreement between you, the end user, and John Wiley & Sons, Inc. ("Wiley"). The enclosed Wiley software program and accompanying data (the "Software") is licensed by Wiley for use only on the terms set forth herein. Please read this license agreement. Registering the product indicates that you accept these terms. If you do not agree to these terms, return the full product (including documentation) with proof of purchase within 30 days for a full refund. In addition, if you are not satisfied with this product for any other reason, you may return the entire product (including documentation) with proof of purchase within 15 days for a full refund.

1. **License:** Wiley hereby grants you, and you accept, a non-exclusive and non-transferable license, to use the Software on the following terms and conditions only:

    (a) The Software is for your personal use only.

    (b) You may use the Software on a single terminal connected to a single computer (i.e., single CPU) and a laptop or other secondary machine for personal use.

    (c) A backup copy or copies of the Software may be made solely for your personal use. Except for such backup copy or copies, you may not copy, modify, distribute, transmit or otherwise reproduce the Software or related documentation, in whole or in part, or systematically store such material in any form or media in a retrieval system; or store such material in electronic format in electronic reading rooms; or transmit such material, directly or indirectly, for use in any service such as document delivery or list serve, or for use by any information brokerage or for systematic distribution of material, whether for a fee or free of charge. You agree to protect the Software and documentation from unauthorized use, reproduction, or distribution.

(d) You agree not to remove or modify any copyright or proprietary notices, author attribution or disclaimer contained in the Software or documentation or on any screen display, and not to integrate material from there with other material or otherwise create derivative works in any medium based on or including materials from the Software or documentation.

(e) You agree not to translate, decompile, disassemble or otherwise reverse engineer the Software.

2. **Limited Warranty:**

(a) Wiley warrants that this product is free of defects in materials and workmanship under normal use for a period of 60 days from the date of purchase as evidenced by a copy of your receipt. If during the 60-day period a defect occurs, you may return the product. Your sole and exclusive remedy in the event of a defect is expressly limited to the replacement of the defective product at no additional charge.

(b) The limited warranty set forth above is in lieu of any and all other warranties, both express and implied, including but not limited to the implied warranties of merchantability or fitness for a particular purpose. The liability of Wiley pursuant to this limited warranty will be limited to replacement of the defective copies of the Software. Some states do not allow the exclusion of implied warranties, so the preceding exclusion may not apply to you.

(c) Because software is inherently complex and may not be completely free of errors, you are advised to verify your work and to make backup copies. In no event will Wiley, nor anyone else involved in creating, producing or delivering the Software, documentation or the materials contained therein, be liable to you for any direct, indirect, incidental, special, consequential or punitive damages arising out of the use or inability to use the Software, documentation or materials contained therein even if advised of the possibility of such damages, or for any claim by any other party. In no case will Wiley's liability exceed the amount paid by you for the Software. Some states do not allow the exclusion or limitation of liability for incidental or consequential damages, so the above limitation or exclusion may not apply to you.

(d) Wiley reserves the right to make changes, additions, and improvements to the Software at any time without notice to any person or organization. No guarantee is made that future versions of the Software will be compatible with any other version.

3. **Term:** Your license to use the Software and documentation will automatically terminate if you fail to comply with the terms of this Agreement. If this license is terminated you agree to destroy all copies of the Software and documentation.

4. **Ownership:** You acknowledge that all rights (including without limitation, copyrights, patents and trade secrets) in the Software and documentation (including without limitation, the structure, sequence, organization, flow, logic, source code, object code and all means and forms of operation of the Software) are the sole and exclusive property of Wiley and/or its licensors, and are protected by the United States copyright laws, other applicable copyright laws, and international treaty provisions.

5. **Restricted Rights:** This Software and/or user documentation are provided with restricted and limited rights. Use, duplication, or disclosure by the Government is subject to restrictions as set forth in paragraph (b)(3)(B) of the Rights in Technical Data and Computer Software clause in DAR 7-104.9(a), FAR 52.2227-14 (June 1987) Alternate III(g)(3)(June 1987), FAR 52.227-19 (June 1987), or DFARS 52.227-701 (c)(1)(ii)(June 1988), or their successors, as applicable. Contractor/manufacturer is John Wiley & Sons, Inc., 111 River Street, Hoboken, NJ 07030.

6. **Canadian Purchase:** If you purchased this product in Canada, you agree to the following: the parties hereto confirm that it is their wish that this Agreement, as well as all other documents relating hereto, including Notices, have been and will be drawn up in the English language only.

7. **Technical Support:** Wiley will respond to all technical support inquiries within 48 hours.

8. **General:** This Agreement represents the entire agreement between us and supersedes any proposals or prior Agreements, oral or written, and any other communication between us relating to the subject matter of this Agreement. This Agreement will be construed and interpreted pursuant to the laws of the State of New York, without regard to such State's conflict of law rules. Any legal action, suit or proceeding arising out of or relating to this Agreement or the breach thereof will be instituted in a court of competent jurisdiction in New York County in the State of New York and each party hereby consents and submits to the personal jurisdiction of such court, waives any objection to venue in such court and consents to the service of process by registered or certified mail, return receipt requested, at the last known address of such party. Should you have any questions concerning this Agreement or if you desire to contact Wiley for any reason, please write to: John Wiley & Sons, Inc., Customer Sales and Service, 111 River Street, Hoboken, NJ 07030.

Index

A
Add-on modules, 5–6, 75
Address labels, 95–97
Administrative reports, 95–98
Aftercare plans, 82–83
Amendments screen, 79–80
Appointment scheduling, 85–88, 129
Approach screen, 64–66
Assessment screens:
   mental status, 50–53
   psychosocial history, 45–46
   recovery, 52–53
   strengths/weaknesses data, 46–47
   summary info, 54
   test/evaluation records, 47–50

B
Billing issues, 73, 74
Blank fields, 21

C
Care level, 63
Case load reports, 97
Check boxes, system, 126–129
Clinical pathways, 24–27, 56
Clinical records reports, 91–95
Custom fields screen, 111
Customization, Thera*Scribe*:
   personal data fields, 42–43
   reports-related, 93–94, 98
   of screens, 4
   session-related fields, 78–79
   tools group choices, 105–106

D
Data analysis:
   patient records, 124–126
   results-oriented, 99–103
Database, 117–126
   backup of, 118–119
   deactivating Thera*Scribe*, 120
   password issues, 119
   TheraSync, 120–126
Dates:
   appointment-related, 86
   entering, 22

Default settings screen, 111–112
Definitions screen, 58–59
Diagnoses:
   data input, 66–67
   editing, 3
   history, 96, 97
Discharge screen, 81–83
Disclosure requests, 126–127
Dropdown lists, 21–22

E
Editing functions:
   assessments, 46–47, 49–50
   attached files, 42
   clinical pathways templates, 26
   diagnoses, 3
   libraries, 29–30, 113–114
   patient records, 79–80
   reports, 4
   treatment plan library, 56, 115–116
Enterprise Edition:
   customization, 30
   installation, 10–13
   login, 16–17

Error files, 129
Essential Edition, 9, 16
Exiting TheraScribe, 34
Exporting data. See Import/export data

F
Fields, 20–21
File menu, 18
Follow-up care. See Aftercare plans

G
General observations screen, 50–51
Goals screen, 59–60
Go menu, 18

H
Help menu, 18–19
HIPAA information:
 data screen, 43–44
 downloading forms, 17
 editing, 114
 in progress notes, 77, 79–80
 security for, 4, 79
Home screen, 17–18, 129
Homework planning, 6, 25, 68–70

I
Import/export data:
 add-on modules, 13
 database management, 117–120
 reports, 89–91, 94–95
Insurance data, 39–40, 128

J
Jongsma, Arthur E., Jr., 1

L
Libraries:
 editing, 29–30, 113–116
 selecting, 28–29, 57–58
Licensing agreement, 133–135
Locking feature, progress notes, 71–72, 79, 127
Log folder, 129
Login names, 108
Login screen, 15–17

M
Mailing labels. See Address labels
Maintenance user check box, 128
Medication-related data, 64–66
Mental status screen, 20, 50–52
Modality screen, 62–64

N
Narrative fields, 21
Navigation bars, 19–20, 35

O
Objective rating screen, 77–78
Objectives/interventions screen, 60–62
Outcomes screens, 99–103
 results, 102–103
 selection criteria, 100–102

P
Passwords, 108–109
Patient records. See also Personal data screens
 amending, 22–24, 79–80
 analysis of, 124–126
 personal data, 37–44
PEC Technologies, 1, 93

Personal data screens:
 attachments, 41–42
 customized data, 42–43
 demographics, 37–39
 general notes, 41
 HIPAA-related, 43–44
 insurance, 39–40
 provider info, 39
Preferences, setting, 129
Problem screen, 56–58
Prognosis/discharge screens, 81–83
Progress notes, 74–77
 customizing, 116–117
 restricting access to, 71–72, 79, 127
Progress screens:
 amendments, 79–80
 customizing data, 78–79
 locking feature, 71–72, 79, 127
 notes planner libraries, 74–77
 objective rating, 77–78
 psychotherapy notes, 78
 session details, 72–74
Provider data, 39, 87–88, 95, 106–110
Psychosocial history, 20, 45–46
Psychotherapy notes, 78

R
Records, patient. See Patient records
Recovery assessment, 52–54
Reports:
 administrative, 89, 95–98
 clinical records, 89, 91–95
 exporting/importing, 89–91
Reports screens, 89–98

Response screen, 67–68
Results analysis. *See* Data analysis
Risk assessment, 52

S
Saving data, 34
Saving screen settings, 33
Scheduling appointments. *See* Appointment scheduling
Screens, customizing, 4, 30–33
Security features:
　HIPAA-related, 4, 79
　progress notes, 71–72, 79, 127
　provider-related, 17, 106–108
　time-out function, 128–129
Session custom fields screen, 78–79
Session data report, 91
Session details screen, 72–74
Sessions date filter, 92
Shortcut bar, 20, 112–113
Small Practice Edition:
　customization features, 30
　installation, 9–10
　login, 16–17
Synchronizing software systems, 120–126
System requirements, 7
System settings, 126–129

T
Tab bars, 20
Teams/groups screen, 110
Testing/evaluation data, 47–50
Therapist Helper, 120–124
Thera*Scribe*:
　activating, 6–7
　Administrator, 106, 107
　capabilities of, 3–5
　contacting, 5–7, 131
　deactivating, 120
　Enterprise Edition, 10–13, 16–17, 30
　Essential Edition, 9, 16
　hardware specs, 7
　installation, 7–13
　licensing agreement, 133–135
　online newsletter, 6
　Small Practice Edition, 9–10, 16–17, 30
　technical support, 131
　Therapist Helper, 120–124
　Trial Edition, 9, 15, 17
TheraSync, 120–126
Thought assessment screen, 51
Tools:
　custom fields screen, 111
　database screen, 117–126
　default settings screen, 111–112
　libraries, 113–114
　overview, 105–106
　preferences, 129
　progress notes screen, 116–117
　providers screen, 106–110
　shortcut bar, 112–113
　system settings screen, 126–129
　teams/groups screen, 110–111
　treatment planners screen, 114–116
Tracking information, 4
Treatment plan screens:
　approach, 64–66
　customizing, 114–116
　definitions, 58–59
　diagnosis, 66–67
　goals, 59–60
　homework, 68–70
　modality, 62–64
　objectives/interventions, 60–62
　overview, 55–56
　problems, 56–58
　response, 67–68
Trial Edition, 9, 15, 17

W
Websites:
　PEC Technologies, 93
　Thera*Scribe,* 5–6, 93